Fibroids

The Latest Treatment Options for this Common Problem

Felicity Smart
Medical Adviser: Professor Stuart Campbell

Thorsons
An Imprint of HarperCollins*Publishers*

Thorsons
An Imprint of HarperCollins*Publishers*
77-85 Fulham Palace Road,
Hammersmith, London W6 8JB

Published by Thorsons 1993
10 9 8 7 6 5 4 3 2 1

© Felicity Smart 1993

Felicity Smart asserts the moral right to
be identified as the author of this work

Illustrations produced by the Department of
Audio Visual Services at Guy's Hospital, London
Artists: Susanna Nasskau and Despina Savva

A catalogue record for this book
is available from the British Library

ISBN 0 7225 2801 9

Typeset by Harper Phototypesetters Limited,
Northampton, England
Printed in Great Britain by
HarperCollinsManufacturing Glasgow

Contents

Foreword

Women today are increasingly aware of their right to choose, and medicine can now offer a much wider range of techniques for treating women's health problems. Fibroids are a very common problem affecting women mainly when in their thirties and forties, although some younger women develop them too. Until quite recently, the treatment for these benign growths in the wall of the womb was limited both by the techniques available and by the attitude of some gynaecologists. Hysterectomy - a major operation to remove the entire womb - was frequently considered to be the most appropriate treatment for large and troublesome fibroids, except for younger women who wanted to have children. Removing the fibroids by performing a myomectomy and reconstructing the womb (another major procedure) was not generally considered necessary or worthwhile for older women.

Now, not only is a greater choice of procedures becoming available (some of which are minor for the patient), but there is also growing acceptance among gynaecologists that a woman's attitude to her body, and to her fertility, must be respected whatever her age. She is entitled to the treatment which she feels is right for her. For some women, that treatment may be a procedure which preserves their womb, while others may still opt for a hysterectomy. But in order to exercise their choice most effectively in their own interests, women need to be well-informed - which is where this book can be particularly helpful. It is the first devoted entirely to the subject of fibroids and it will therefore enable women to gain a much better understanding of this problem and of the possible treatments. Most importantly, it will also make it far easier for a woman with troublesome fibroids to discuss the treatment options with her gynaecologist and arrive at an informed choice. This is a needed and most welcome book.

In addition, the book will contribute to fundraising for the new Research Centre for Women's Health, which I am establishing at King's College Hospital. The Centre will coordinate research, education, screening and treatment programmes concerning every aspect of the mature woman's health - thus pioneering for a healthier future for women everywhere.

PROFESSOR STUART CAMPBELL
Head of Obstetrics and Gynaecology
King's College Hospital, London

Acknowledgements

We thank the following for their contributions to the writing of this book:

Mr S L Tan, Senior Lecturer and Consultant, Department of Obstetrics and Gynaecology, King's College Hospital, London;

Mr Thomas Bourne, Lecturer, Department of Obstetrics and Gynaecology, King's College Hospital, London;

Dr N Whitelaw, Research Registrar, The Royal Surrey County Hospital;

Rosemary Conley and The Evening Standard for permission to quote from 'Me And My Health'.

Felicity Smart personally thanks Diana Bowen-Jones for the introduction to Professor Campbell; Joy Langridge, who always helps; Jane Graham-Maw, Editorial Director at Thorsons, for keeping the whole show going; Veronica Simpson, for her editorial advice; Sue Ferguson Linnell, who always encourages; Nicola Williams, for patiently word-processing many drafts; Tim Smart, husband and life-support.

Acknowledgment

Introduction

Having been successfully treated for fibroids myself, this book is very much the result of personal experience. I was diagnosed as having these benign growths in my womb at a routine check-up. As a general medical editor and writer, I knew what they were and how they could be treated. Fibroids can enlarge and distort the womb, they can cause unpleasant symptoms, impair fertility, and may require surgery. I'd had vague symptoms, but hadn't related them to this problem. It therefore came as a shock when my doctor told me that my fibroids were already large and could continue to grow, and so needed treatment.

Although I had some knowledge, I still read everything I could find on fibroids, looking for more information and reassurance. I discovered that there was little detailed advice given, compared to the very much larger amount available on other common health problems. It's estimated that the number of women affected by fibroids is as many as one in four, and may possibly be more. Most often fibroids occur when women have reached what enlightened doctors describe as 'the later reproductive years'. They are also found in some who are younger. Yet there wasn't a book for women devoted entirely to the subject.

I was referred to a gynaecologist - and became a recent example of the situation Professor Campbell has described in his foreword. Without hesitation, I was recommended to have a hysterectomy to remove my womb. This was a further shock as I had thought that a myomectomy - an operation which removes the fibroids only and restores the womb to normal -

would be an option. But no; given my age (I was in my late thirties), my womb and I were considered to have had our best years together. There would be little point in restoring my fertility now.

I explained (it wasn't easy) that for me, having a womb was not simply a matter of fertility. I regarded my womb as an important part of myself as a woman. Since there could be a choice of treatment for fibroids, I didn't want my womb to be removed. I saw nothing wrong with keeping my fertility either. This attitude was not seen as sensible. Fortunately, even in the relatively short time since that consultation, there has been increasing recognition among doctors and gynaecologists that whatever a woman's feelings, she must be allowed to influence the proposed treatment.

We can view ourselves in such different ways: for some women with problem fibroids, restoring their fertility will be crucial, while for others this may not be the priority. A perfect example of how a hysterectomy can be a very positive choice is given in this book by Rosemary Conley, the glamorous British author famous for her bestsellers on diet and fitness. What matters most, however, is that we are informed of the possible treatments and feel free to discuss them with our gynaecologist, so that we can make the decision which is right for us as individuals.

My own story has a happy ending. I decided that I needed a second opinion (don't hesitate to ask your doctor to refer you to another specialist, if you think it necessary). But I was also attending a Yoga class, and this was to help in unexpected ways. It was through Yoga that I met Diana Bowen-Jones, the friend who introduced me to Professor Stuart Campbell. He completely understood the need to discuss my problem fully and sympathetically, which resulted in my having the myomectomy.

Fibroids are certainly an underrated problem, which is why I have written this book, the first solely dedicated to them. Professor Campbell has given me much invaluable help and advice. We explain what fibroids are, their symptoms, the treatments and how best to cope with them. Major surgery, such as I had, is an option for troublesome fibroids, but now drugs combined with new procedures which are minor for the woman may be offered.

Facing hospital treatment can be very frightening, even when it is for a benign problem. We have therefore advised on preparing for treatment, given information and reassurance on what to expect in hospital, and shown how you can speed recovery. I found that Yoga relaxation techniques were a great help throughout, and so I've included several methods of keeping calm and relaxed which you may find helpful.

Being calm and well-informed gives you confidence. This book is here to provide women with all the necessary information. For those needing treatment, we hope it will contribute to a positive outcome based on the best decision.

FELICITY SMART

CHAPTER ONE
What Are Fibroids?

A fibroid is a growth which can develop within, or from, the wall of the womb. Don't be alarmed by the word 'growth' (which means the same as a lump or tumour) when it's used to describe a fibroid. When fibroids occur - and there is usually more than one - they are virtually always benign. This means they are non-cancerous. Fibroids can sometimes grow large; they can cause unpleasant symptoms and other problems which need medical treatment, but they are not normally life-threatening. If you've been diagnosed as having fibroids, however, or are concerned that you might be developing them, you are likely to want information and reassurance on what is happening to your womb - and about any treatment which may be necessary.

It's worth mentioning at the start of the book that doctors often refer to the womb by its Latin name of 'uterus'. You may already be familiar with the term, but there have been cases where patients thought some other organ was being discussed because the word 'womb' wasn't used by their doctor. For the same reason, it's also worth knowing that the medical term for a fibroid is 'uterine myoma' or 'fibromyoma'. 'Myomata' or 'fibromyomata' therefore mean more than one fibroid. They may also be referred to as 'leiomyoma/leiomyomata', which mean the same things, although most doctors do call them fibroids.

The Structure of Fibroids

What exactly are they? In its normal state, the womb is about the size and shape of a small pear. Most of it is muscle and this enables it to contract during labour so that the baby can be born. It can contract at other times, such as during periods - a reason why they may be painful - and pleasurably during orgasm. Fibroids develop within, or from, this muscular wall.

The womb itself is pinkish-grey and fibroids appear as whitish lumps, contained in a fibrous pouch or capsule. They are made of solid, hard bundles of fibrous and muscular tissue. They differ from cancerous tumours because the cells from which they are made still have the same structure as normal womb cells, and they grow in a more controlled manner. In contrast, cancerous cells don't resemble the cells of the organ from which they grow - and they multiply in a dangerous, haywire way. Cancerous tumours can grow beyond themselves and invade surrounding healthy tissue; cells can break off from them and spread round the body to form malignant growths elsewhere. Fibroids, however, remain self-contained.

They begin by being very small, and may remain so, but - as has already been mentioned - they can sometimes grow large. Their size is often compared to fruit and vegetables because they can vary from very tiny, like seeds, to pea-sized, through tomato and orange, to very large: grapefruit or melon-sized. They can cause the womb to become bulky and misshapen, but they are almost always slow-growing and take years to develop. Just very occasionally, a large fibroid may turn into a cancerous tumour called a sarcoma, but it would most likely have caused symptoms by then and been treated.

Inside the womb there is a cavity, or space, which has a lining called the endometrium. Throughout a woman's fertile life this lining is prepared during the menstrual cycle to receive a fertilized egg, so that a pregnancy can be started. When there is no fertilized egg, the endometrium is shed as a period. The womb lining is then renewed and the menstrual cycle continues until it is interrupted by a pregnancy, or when periods and fertility cease at the menopause. Hormones control the menstrual cycle by acting as 'chemical messengers'. One of these hormones is called oestrogen; how its role may relate to the development of fibroids is discussed later on p 20.

Sites of Fibroids

Fibroids can cause a variety of symptoms and need different treatments, depending on their sites, so it will be helpful if we describe them.

Intramural fibroids grow within the muscular wall of the womb. If they grow large, the womb itself increases in size.

Subserous fibroids grow from the outer wall of the womb into the abdomen, sometimes on a stalk. These too can become large.

Submucous fibroids grow from the inner wall of the womb, just under the endometrium. They can sometimes protrude into the cavity on a stalk, although this kind doesn't usually enlarge quite as much as fibroids in other sites because it is further away from the main blood supply.

A fibroid which grows on a stalk is known medically as a **pedunculated fibroid** (a peduncle being the connecting stalk). Very rarely, a pedunculated subserous fibroid may become what is know as a **parasitic fibroid**. This can happen if the stalk twists, cutting off the fibroid's blood supply. The fibroid then attaches itself to another organ in the pelvis, such as the bowel, and takes its blood supply from it. Far more often though, a fibroid which loses its blood supply degenerates, causing the symptoms described later on p 27.

Fibroids less commonly grow on or in the cervix, which is the womb's entrance/exit, often called 'the neck of the womb'. (This is the round pad of flesh which can be felt with your finger at the top of your vagina.) They generally affect the main body of the womb. But a pedunculated submucous fibroid may occasionally protrude on its stalk through the cervix into the vagina, having been pushed out by contractions of the womb. It can enlarge in the vagina. Sometimes the womb doesn't succeed in pushing it right out and it becomes stuck in the cervix. Unpleasant symptoms can result in both such cases (see chapter 3).

We have said earlier that a woman with fibroids is likely to have more than one, and they may also be of different sizes and in various sites, as illustrated on the next page.

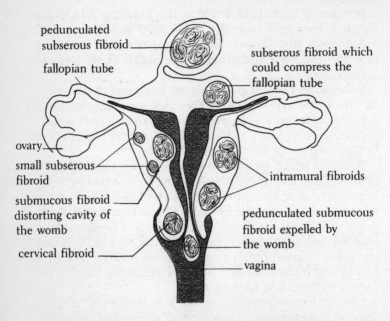

pedunculated
subserous fibroid

fallopian tube

subserous fibroid which
could compress the
fallopian tube

ovary

small subserous
fibroid

submucous fibroid
distorting cavity of
the womb

cervical fibroid

intramural fibroids

pedunculated submucous
fibroid expelled by
the womb

vagina

*A womb showing where fibroids could develop.
In reality, few women would have them in all
these sites.*

Why Do They Occur?

It isn't really known why fibroids occur, but about a quarter of all women develop them, usually when they are in their thirties and forties, before they have been through the menopause. Childless women, and women who had children later in life (rather than in their teens or twenties) are more likely to be affected. Although younger women generally are much less likely to have them, there are exceptions; black women are also prone to getting them in their late teens and twenties. Why this should be so isn't known either.

It does appear, however, that high levels of the female hormone oestrogen - referred to in the previous chapter - influence their growth, even though it's not thought to be the actual cause. To explain this hormone's role, we'll describe how it is produced, and what it does, during the menstrual cycle.

The Menstrual Cycle

An area of the brain, called the hypothalamus, co-ordinates our hormonal and nervous systems. This small area, no larger than an olive, is situated behind the eyes and connects with the even smaller pituitary gland below it at the base of the brain. The pituitary receives instructions from the hypothalamus to release hormones into the bloodstream.

On day one of your menstrual cycle, when a period starts, the pituitary releases a hormone called follicle stimulating hormone (FSH). This hormone travels to the ovaries via the bloodstream. The ovaries are a pair of glands about the size of walnuts situated on either side of the womb, and each ovary is attached to it by a ligament (see the illustration on p 18). The function of the ovaries is to produce eggs for fertilization. FSH, as its name suggests, stimulates one or other of your ovaries to produce follicles (they look like small blisters on the surface of the ovary) in which eggs ripen. This takes from 12-14 days on average.

During this time, the hormone oestrogen is produced by the ovary. This causes the womb lining to grow and thicken. The pituitary gland responds to the oestrogen by producing another hormone, called luteinizing hormone (LH), which causes one of the follicles to burst, releasing the ripe egg on about day 14. This is known as ovulation. The egg is scooped up by the fronds (fimbriae) at the end of the fallopian tube near the ovary. There are two such tubes which connect with the womb, one on each side adjacent to the ovaries. The egg passes slowly down the tube for about three to four days. This is where the egg may be fertilized by a man's sperm, which swims from the vagina, through the cervix, into the womb and up the tube, where it penetrates the egg.

Meanwhile, the empty follicle turns yellow (it's then called the 'corpus luteum' or 'yellow body') and secretes the hormone progesterone; this 'balances' the hormone oestrogen by preparing the womb lining for its function: to receive a fertilized egg and start a pregnancy.

The fertilized egg, now called an embryo, develops for a few days in the fallopian tube and then travels to the womb, where it implants in the lining and becomes a pregnancy. During pregnancy both oestrogen and progesterone production increase and there are high oestrogen levels. If fertilization doesn't happen, levels of oestrogen and progesterone fall and the womb lining comes away as a period on about day 28. Another cycle then starts. This description is based on an average 28-day cycle, but variations in the number of days in any woman's cycle are not unusual or abnormal.

The Oestrogen Connection

Although oestrogen is not thought to cause fibroids, there is evidence that it influences their size. It seems to make some, though not necessarily all, fibroids enlarge; a woman may have a number of fibroids, some of which are tiny while others may vary in size, like the fruit and vegetables mentioned earlier.

The oestrogen connection has been made because fibroids can often enlarge dramatically when oestrogen levels are high, such as when a woman with fibroids becomes pregnant. Conversely, taking the contraceptive pill may reduce the size of fibroids because of the progestogen (synthetic progesterone) content. Both the combined and phased pill contain oestrogen, but this is 'balanced' by the progestogen; the progestogen-only pill, formerly also known as the minipill, contains no oestrogen as its name indicates. It has been suggested that taking the pill might offer some protection against fibroids occurring in the first place. It is not, however, seen as sufficiently effective to be used to shrink fibroids, although it may help to control symptoms (see chapter 5 on Treatments). Drugs which act on the hypothalamus and the pituitary gland to inhibit oestrogen production can shrink fibroids; there is more about them on p 54.

When oestrogen production declines naturally at the menopause, fibroids shrink and may become undetectable, especially if they were small. But if hormone replacement therapy (HRT) is given, it can make them enlarge a bit. This is because oestrogen is being replaced to relieve severe menopausal symptoms, such as hot flushes/flashes and night sweats, which are due to the decline in this hormone. Progestogen is also given in HRT, but not continuously as in the pill. Any troublesome fibroids would have been treated by this time, however, so the possibility of fibroids which have not caused problems becoming a bit bigger wouldn't be a reason for not having HRT. Relieving severe menopausal symptoms which may be making the woman's life a misery would be much more important.

Fibroids in themselves have no effect on hormonal balance at any time. They may respond to hormones by increasing or decreasing in size, but their presence doesn't influence the way in which a woman's hormones behave.

Other Factors

In the absence of further medical evidence, one can only speculate about other factors which may make fibroids develop. A woman with fibroids may well do just that. If she is in her thirties or forties and has no children, or delayed childbearing beyond her twenties, she may wonder whether the fibroids are a sign that her womb has in some way deteriorated because it was denied its reproductive purpose at her most fertile time in life. This is not so. Fibroids are not 'dead' tissue; they have a blood supply. A womb with fibroids will continue to function, even though it may not be problem-free. Or she may think that because her womb has not 'grown' a baby, it has produced something else instead. There is no medical basis for this supposition (see below).

A woman's actual fertility seems to have no connection with fibroids. Women who are childless due to infertility, or who had fertility problems which delayed motherhood, share the same risk of fibroids as fertile women who have not had children early in life. Why early childbearing should apparently give some protection against developing fibroids is unknown, but even if you have children when young it's no absolute guarantee. There are cases of women who've had children early getting fibroids later. And, clearly, there is no such protection for black women, who are prone to fibroids at a young age, often before they've had a chance to start families. Even when they've had children, the positive effect of pregnancy doesn't seem to be so strong in them. Therefore, the idea that fibroids might grow instead of a pregnancy is far from logical, since childbearing is by no means a protection in every case.

Some research shows that very overweight women are more liable to have problems with fibroids. Body fat produces oestrogen independently of the ovaries, so the more fatty tissue there is, the more oestrogen there is likely to be - but slim women who have never been overweight can sometimes develop large fibroids too. However, an overweight woman may well be advised to lose weight by her doctor, especially if she is recommended to have an operation for fibroids; see p 59 for the reasons.

Is stress a factor? This is a question which anyone with a health problem is likely to ask today. There are no clear-cut answers. Stress, anxiety and unhappiness can undermine us in so many ways. Sometimes people may just *feel* they can relate a health problem to stress, however. The hypothalamus - the area of the brain which co-ordinates our hormonal and nervous systems - also registers our emotions. Stress may influence hormonal balance. Although a connection with fibroids is not proven, perhaps it cannot be ruled out either. Certainly, stress and negative emotions are no help to anyone who is coping with treatment for fibroids. We've therefore included advice on relieving stress; see chapter 9 on Self-Help.

CHAPTER THREE
Symptoms

Women with fibroids often have no symptoms: they aren't necessarily related to the size or number of fibroids. However, the more numerous and/or the larger they are, the more likely a woman is to have troublesome symptoms, although small fibroids can sometimes cause problems too.

What symptoms are they likely to cause? The most common one for which women seek medical help is heavy, prolonged periods. This problem is known medically as menorrhagia. They may be experiencing 'flooding' and blood clots; they may also have cramping pains. Heavy periods due to fibroids are not always painful, though. Periods can also be irregular and there may be bleeding between periods, but this is less usual. It dep:nds on where the fibroids are located.

The most troublesome are the submucous fibroids which grow in the muscular wall of the womb, just under the endometrium. They can cause heavier periods in two ways; by enlarging and distorting the cavity of the womb and the endometrium (the area that bleeds), or by increasing the number and size of blood vessels under the lining of the womb. Sometimes they do both. Heavy periods can result in anaemia (iron deficiency) which makes you feel fatigued and depressed.

If a submucous fibroid grows into the cavity on a stalk (a pedunculated submucous fibroid), the womb may treat it as a 'foreign body' and try to push it out through the cervix. This causes cramping pains, like a mini-labour, particularly during periods. If this type of fibroid becomes stuck in the cervix, it can also cause bleeding and pain at other times, such as during and after sex. It may be pushed right out into the vagina where it can enlarge, also causing discomfort and bleeding during and after sex.

It must be emphasized that such symptoms can have causes other than fibroids. If you have any abnormal bleeding, you *must* see your doctor promptly.

As has already been said, fibroids which actually grow on or in the cervix are uncommon. When they are present, they can also cause painful periods by obstructing bleeding.

Intramural fibroids (which grow inside the wall of the womb) and subserous fibroids (they grow from the outer wall, sometimes on a stalk) can both cause the abdomen to swell if they become large. This may be noticeable, like a pregnancy, particularly in a slim woman. There is a lot of room in the pelvis, however, and so the swelling may not be obvious. It may be possible for a woman to feel an enlarged womb, and large pedunculated fibroids, by pressing her abdomen.

These types of fibroids can cause a variety of symptoms, depending on their size and how much pressure they put on other organs. A bulky womb can press on the bladder, resulting in the need to urinate frequently. Large fibroids at the back of the womb at its base can cause the whole womb to tip backwards; its normal position is leaning slightly forwards, though in some women it is naturally tilted backwards, which seldom causes any problems. This is called retroversion and when it happens due to fibroids the cervix can be pushed forwards so that it presses on the neck of the bladder. Urination can be completely cut off. This is not a common problem, but it is serious and requires urgent treatment in hospital. Initially, a catheter (a tube) is inserted into the urethra – the passage through which you urinate – to empty the bladder. The fibroids must then be treated surgically, either by a myomectomy or a hysterectomy; see chapter 6.

Pressure on other organs can cause backache, pelvic discomfort, constipation and even varicose veins, if fibroids press on veins from the legs. Fibroids may cause pelvic discomfort during sex, but this is unusual.

It isn't easy for a woman to relate any such symptoms to fibroids and she may interpret them in a completely different way. Here is how one woman viewed her symptoms prior to a routine check-up with her doctor.

'I'd been wondering why I couldn't hold my stomach in,

but had put it down to flabby muscles. After all, I was in my late thirties and I had a sedentary job. But then hadn't I quit on my jogging because I always seemed to get caught short - another sign of age? Weren't my periods heavier? Yes, but couldn't that be for the same reason?

'Now my doctor was telling me I had large fibroids. The flabby tum in fact housed a swollen womb. When I jogged it had put pressure on my bladder. And, yes, my periods would be heavier with a distorted womb.'

This illustrates just one good reason why it is wise to have regular routine check-ups at the intervals recommended by your doctor or clinic, even if you think nothing is really wrong. There are also other potentially serious problems unrelated to fibroids which have few or no early symptoms, but which can be successfully treated at this stage. This doesn't mean you should worry about being ill even when you feel perfectly well; most women are as healthy as they feel, but even so it is very worthwhile to have regular check-ups simply as a means of protecting and reassuring yourself.

Painful Fibroids

Fibroids are seldom painful, though occasionally they can cause acute pain. This can happen if a pedunculated fibroid twists on its stalk - as already mentioned - cutting off its own blood supply. (A pedunculated fibroid is rather like a weight on the end of a rope and normal movement in the pelvis can cause it to twist.) This is called infarction. In addition to acute pain, the woman may have a fever, feel sick, and have local tenderness when her abdomen is touched. An ultrasound scan (see p 35) would show a pedunculated fibroid and the pain from it would indicate that it had twisted. Although it is a very unpleasant experience, fortunately it rarely happens and the problem is not serious in itself.

Treatment, which would be in hospital, can simply be painkillers and bed rest - with sedation if necessary - while the pain lasts. A fibroid without a blood supply hardens and shrivels into a stone-like lump, called a 'womb stone', which is not harmful and no treatment is needed. However, some specialists may offer to operate and remove an infarcted subserous fibroid in its acutely painful stage. This would involve opening the abdomen under general anaesthetic, clamping the stalk and cutting off the fibroid, which would take no more than 10 minutes to perform. It could be described as an 'easy myomectomy'. Chapter 6 gives a fuller description of how a myomectomy is carried out. If a pedunculated submucous fibroid growing out into the cavity of the womb degenerates, causing acute pain, it could be removed by endometrial ablation or resection, procedures described in chapter 5.

A fibroid can also degenerate during pregnancy, although this too is a very rare occurrence. It can happen because there are high oestrogen levels and a plentiful blood supply to the womb, which may make some fibroids likely to enlarge considerably. These fibroids are more vascular (they have a greater blood supply) than others, which is why they may be affected. As a result of the enlargement, the blood supply can't always reach the centre of the fibroid, which then starts to degenerate and there is bleeding into the fibroid. It is a mixture of infarction and degeneration, called 'red degeneration'.

The symptoms are the same as in infarction. However, there is a risk of miscarriage or premature labour because red degeneration can make the womb contract. A pregnant woman with fibroids should therefore be alert to any cramping pains and go to a hospital as quickly as possible. Drugs can be given either intravenously or by mouth which calm the womb and relieve the pain. After the baby is born, a degenerated fibroid usually shrinks away.

Red degeneration cannot be prevented because it is not possible to treat most fibroids during pregnancy. Pedunculated subserous ones growing from the outer wall could be removed by 'easy myomectomy', which might be done if they degenerated in pregnancy, although many surgeons would consider removal unnecessary. Surgery of all kinds should be avoided if possible during pregnancy. Fibroids which grow elsewhere within the womb cannot be treated while the woman is pregnant. As red degeneration is such a rare occurrence, however, the risk of miscarriage is small. Nevertheless, if you are thinking of becoming pregnant and know you have fibroids, it's worth having a check-up, and any treatment considered necessary, before conceiving. Colour ultrasound can show the blood flow to a fibroid, and this can indicate whether red degeneration is likely to happen. But it is so rare that, after the risks have been assessed, a woman may be advised to go ahead and become pregnant anyway. Fibroids and pregnancy often co-exist without problems.

Fibroids and Fertility

Do fibroids ever actually prevent conception? Is infertility therefore ever a symptom of fibroids? They are not a major cause of infertility: there are much more likely to be other reasons why a woman is having difficultly conceiving. But if fibroids block the fallopian tubes, so that sperm can't get through to fertilize the egg in the tube, they will prevent conception, although this problem seldom arises.

Fibroids which grow out into the cavity of the womb may act rather like the IUD (intra-uterine device), a contraceptive which is inserted into the womb and prevents an embryo from implanting. They also take up space within the womb, which can make it difficult for a pregnancy to continue.

A 'womb stone' (see p 27) is not usually a problem, mainly because a woman is likely to be past childbearing age by the time it develops.

Miscarriage is not often caused by fibroids, but there are a few situations in which it may occur. If an embryo implants directly on top of a submucous fibroid in the wall of the womb, it may not attach itself very well and so come away as an early miscarriage. We have already described red degeneration. A womb which is very misshapen or enlarged by fibroids may also be unable to sustain a pregnancy. But even if your womb were so distorted by fibroids that childbearing would be impossible, you may be able to have a myomectomy (see chapter 6), the operation which removes fibroids and restores the womb to normal.

Lastly, large fibroids which grow in or on the cervix blocking the exit (they're uncommon) will interfere with childbirth. A natural birth would not be possible, and the baby would have to be born by Caesarean delivery: via an incision in the abdomen.

CHAPTER FOUR

Diagnosing Fibroids

Because fibroids often have no symptoms – or cause symptoms which are difficult for a woman to interpret – diagnosis is frequently made during a routine check-up. Or she may have consulted her doctor for some other gynaecological problem, which may or may not be related to fibroids. We have already said how important it is to have regular check-ups, and to see your doctor about any symptoms. When you make an appointment with your doctor or at a clinic, ensure that you won't be having a period at the time.

The most usual way in which a doctor begins diagnosing fibroids is simply by feeling the abdomen. You need undress only below the waist and lie comfortably on the examination couch with your knees bent and your feet apart. A sheet or blanket covers your lower body, but you can remove it if you want to see more of what is happening.

The doctor starts by gently pressing the abdomen by hand (called palpation) to feel for anything unusual. Even quite small fibroids can sometimes be felt through the abdominal wall. A bimanual (two-handed) pelvic examination will also be carried out. The doctor slips one or two fingers, which have been lubricated, into the vagina and again presses the abdomen gently with the other hand, as illustrated. This enables the womb and ovaries to be felt. The doctor can feel the size of the womb and get a clearer idea of the fibroids' position. It helps if you are not overweight, as it is more difficult to feel the pelvic organs through a thick layer of fat. The examination should not hurt, although the ovaries can be sensitive when handled, as can the womb when the cervix is

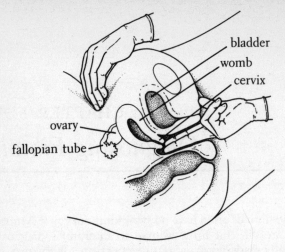

bladder
womb
cervix
ovary
fallopian tube

A womb enlarged or distorted by fibroids would be felt during a routine bimanual (two-handed) pelvic examination.

moved. Say immediately if you feel any pain.

A routine check-up will include a breast examination and a cervical smear test. This simple, painless procedure removes a few cells from the cervix for testing to ensure there are no early changes related to cervical cancer (called pre-cancerous changes). The results most often show that everything is normal. If there are any pre-cancerous changes, they can be completely cured, so the test is always worth doing. For more information on how a full check-up is carried out, we recommend you to read the chapter on Diagnosing Women's Problems in *The Woman's Guide To Surgery* (Thorsons).

If you have small fibroids which aren't causing trouble, no treatment is needed, but your doctor will want to check them at intervals to see if they are enlarging. You should ensure that you do see your doctor for them to be monitored. It isn't necessary to remove these fibroids simply because they might cause trouble later. Surgery to the womb weakens it, which may mean that if you then have a baby, a normal delivery could be inadvisable and you would need a Caesarean. As has already been said, fibroids don't necessarily interfere with pregnancy.

For fibroids which are enlarged and/or causing trouble, you

will be referred to a gynaecologist - a specialist in problems of the female reproductive system. The gynaecologist will want to examine you again, as just described, and may carry out other diagnostic procedures. Gynaecologists are also surgeons and will therefore perform any procedures or treatments needing surgery. But if you are referred to a gynaecologist, this doesn't mean that you will automatically be 'under the knife'.

Resolving Anxieties

Before we say any more about diagnosing fibroids, some words of advice may help those women who are worried about having a check-up and seeing a gynaecologist.

The possibility of having a health problem needing treatment can actually deter some women from seeking medical advice, even though it is obviously the sensible thing to do. They may fear finding out that something is wrong and the disruption treatment could cause to their lives, so they'd rather not know. They may persuade themselves that they are just 'too busy' to bother right now.

In addition, doctors and specialists are often perceived as figures of authority; patients can sometimes feel overawed and intimidated by them, particularly at a first consultation. But your body is owned by you, not by the medical profession, and the choice to have any treatment is entirely yours. Their role is to advise you and make recommendations as to the best course of treatment.

Understanding what is wrong, and how treatment can resolve the problem, will help you to feel more confident - which is where this book comes in if you have fibroids. The information and advice given here should enable you to communicate better with your doctor and gynaecologist.

If, however, you find you simply can't get on with a particular doctor, you should change to another. At a clinic, you can ask to see someone else. Similarly, your doctor can refer you to another gynaecologist if necessary. Any such difficulties do not necessarily mean that a doctor or gynaecologist is less good medically, but it is important to be able to relax and talk openly.

For some women, another source of anxiety and

embarrassment about having a pelvic examination can be that the doctor or gynaecologist is a man (the majority still are men, although an increasing number now are women); he may also be a stranger. A female nurse may be present during the examination, although this is not always the case. You can ask for one to be there. Or you can ask to see a woman doctor if you are attending a clinic where there are several doctors, but you would need to do this in advance and it may not be possible. Your doctor may be able to refer you to a woman gynaecologist, though you might have to accept a man. But some women feel just as awkward with a woman doctor or gynaecologist.

Such feelings may sometimes actually arise more from a woman's own fears of having a check-up at all. A friendly, sympathetic doctor - whether male or female - can often dispel them. You can take a partner, relative or friend with you, if you think this will help. Sometimes, however, it can in fact be easier to speak freely if you go on your own.

Talking to other patients prior to a consultation can be reassuring. And an excellent self-help method of reducing anxiety, which can be carried out while you are waiting, is to take several deep breaths, concentrating on breathing out slowly (see chapter 9 on Self-Help for more on relaxation techniques).

You don't have to undress in front of the doctor or gynaecologist. Either s/he will leave the room, or you can go behind a curtain or screen. At a clinic, you may be asked to undress beforehand and put on the gown provided.

Remember that doctors and gynaecologists are professionals and won't judge or criticize you. They're also very used to carrying out check-ups and a woman's most personal anatomy is a familiar sight to them. Many today are aware of patients' anxieties and will try to reassure you, and will explain what they are doing. If you need more information, don't hesitate to ask.

Diagnostic Procedures

The procedures which may be used in diagnosis are as follows. After the gynaecologist has examined you, s/he will recommend those which are appropriate, should they be necessary.

A **blood test** will show whether heavy periods have caused anaemia. This just involves removing a blood sample by syringe from a vein in your arm for testing. Hormone levels can also be checked from a blood sample. Towards the menopause, they may indicate how much longer your periods are likely to continue, which could influence the choice of treatment.

An **ultrasound scan** enables fibroids to be seen (scanned) to confirm their size and position. This diagnostic procedure is completely painless and there is little discomfort. It is carried out at a clinic or hospital on an out-patient basis, which means that you can go home straight after. Ultrasound is considered to be safe and there are no known after-effects.

There are two methods of carrying out the scan; it can be done abdominally or via the vagina, and takes only about fifteen minutes, or less.

With abdominal ultrasound, you need to have a full bladder because this separates the pelvic organs, making them easier to see. If you're not already in this state, you will be given a jug of water and a glass and be asked to drink as much as you can.

You don't have to undress, just push your clothes down over your hips. Oil or jelly is then applied to your abdomen (this won't stain your skin or clothes and is simply wiped off after the procedure). It ensures that the instrument used by the doctor, called a transducer, has maximum contact and will move easily on your skin. The transducer is moved slowly over your abdomen above your womb. What it does is to bounce high-frequency sound waves (too high to be heard) off your pelvic organs and then translate them into images on a video monitor, as illustrated. It's fascinating to watch; the doctor will explain the images on view.

Trans-vaginal ultrasound is being used increasingly because it gives better pictures, particularly of troublesome fibroids under the endometrium. You don't need a full bladder, but you will need to undress below the waist. You then sit or lie on the examination couch with your feet supported apart by stirrups. This method uses a probe as a transducer, which is covered by a lubricated condom and inserted into the vagina to pick up

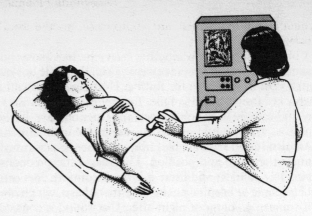

Abdominal ultrasound is a completely painless procedure which shows the size and position of fibroids on a video monitor.

the images. It fits easily and is moved around a bit, which is only slightly uncomfortable.

Ultrasound images can be in black and white or include colour. With more advanced machines, you will be able to see streaks of colour superimposed on the black and white pictures. This is called colour doppler and works on the principle that blood flowing within the vessels will send back signals at a changed frequency, depending on the speed of blood flow. It therefore gives a colour picture of the blood vessels in the womb and surrounding organs. The blood flow in a fibroid can be seen in colour, as mentioned earlier, and this indicates whether or not the fibroid is likely to enlarge. During pregnancy, both fetus and fibroids can be monitored by ultrasound.

Hysteroscopy allows the gynaecologist to look directly inside the womb. It is quite a new procedure which is carried out using a hysteroscope. This is a small viewing instrument about 1 cm (½ in) in diameter, which is inserted into the womb via the cervix under anaesthetic, so you don't feel anything. It has a light and a lens at one end, and there can be several channels in it: one for looking down, another through which fluid or gas can be passed into the womb to separate the walls and give a better view, and there can be a channel through which fine instruments can be inserted into the womb for minor surgery.

It enables the gynaecologist to see whether heavy periods are caused by small fibroids growing into the cavity, or by very small polyps, which don't show up on ultrasound (although larger ones can be seen). These are benign lumps which grow on a stalk from the membrane lining the womb, and they can also grow from the cervix into the vagina. They are not as large as fibroids, but can cause similar menstrual symptoms, bleeding between periods and after sex. They are often associated with fibroids and so a woman may have both, but polyps alone would not produce other problems, as do fibroids. The internal openings of the fallopian tubes into the cavity can also be seen by hysteroscopy and assessed for possible blockage.

When hysteroscopy is used simply to take a look, it can be done on an out-patient basis under sedation and a local anaesthetic; this is injected into the cervix and hurts only momentarily. There are no after-effects and you can go home quite soon following the procedure (but do arrange for transport, as you shouldn't drive straight away). More often, however, it is combined with other procedures.

Some gynaecologists may recommend a procedure called an HSG (see p 85) and/or a laparoscopy (p 40) to assess the fibroids' position, but others may rely on ultrasound and hysteroscopy.

D & C (dilation/dilatation and curettage) is not exactly a diagnostic procedure for fibroids, but it may be used to ensure that fibroids - or polyps - and not something else, are responsible for abnormal bleeding. Its purpose is to biopsy (remove) samples of the womb lining for examination under a microscope. It is one of the most common minor surgical procedures and is needed by the majority of women at some time in their lives. One of its uses is to diagnose cancerous changes, but if you are having a D & C, it doesn't necessarily mean you have cancer. Benign causes of abnormal bleeding are far more likely, but it is the major reason why you must not delay reporting any such symptoms.

At most, a D & C requires only an overnight stay in hospital but it can often be carried out on a day-patient basis (you are

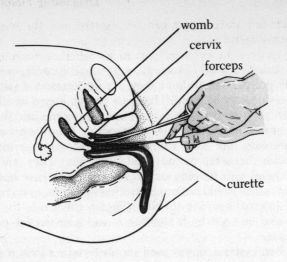

womb
cervix
forceps
curette

Removing samples of womb lining by D & C
(dilation and curettage) for examination can
determine whether or not fibroids are causing
heavy periods.

in hospital only for the day). It is usually done under a general anaesthetic; for information about procedures carried out under general anaesthetic, see pp 65-69. A local anaesthetic can be used, however, and this will be injected into the cervix. The vagina is held open using an instrument called a speculum, so the cervix can be seen. It needs to be widened (dilated) to allow the womb lining to be removed. The cervix is therefore steadied with forceps so that metal or plastic rods (dilators) of increasing size can be inserted to dilate it. These are removed and a spoon-shaped instrument called a curette is then passed into the womb so the endometrium can be gently scraped, as illustrated. This is why a D & C is often called 'a scrape'. The whole procedure takes only about 10 minutes to perform.

It can be used to remove polyps and may be combined with a hysteroscopy. As already described, hysteroscopy enables polyps in the womb to be located; they can then be removed by D & C, and the gynaecologist can check again afterwards using the hysteroscope to see whether the procedure has been successful. If necessary, forceps can be passed down a channel in the hysteroscope to biopsy samples of the womb lining.

Following a D & C you may have some bleeding and mild period-like cramps for a day or two. Sanitary towels, not tampons, should be used, because tampons increase the risk of infection. This is a hazard of surgical procedures involving the womb, cervix and vagina. It is not due to any medical negligence, but can occur because the vagina can't be completely sterilized; it is open to the air, in which bacteria are always present. Should there be any infection - signs of which are a smelly discharge and cramping pains - it can be successfully treated with antibiotics.

Don't have sex until bleeding stops. Your periods may be irregular for a month or two afterwards, until the womb lining returns to normal, but use contraception right away unless you want to become pregnant. Most women resume their normal lives the day after a D & C and the procedure has no long-term effects.

Suction curettage is being increasingly used to biopsy the womb lining to find out the causes of abnormal bleeding. It can be done without any anaesthetic and so is an out-patient procedure. It simply involves inserting a very fine metal or plastic tube into the womb via the cervix, which doesn't need to be dilated beforehand. Samples of womb lining are removed by applying low pressure vacuum suction to the tube. It takes a few minutes to perform and can occasionally be slightly uncomfortable. The after-effects are milder than a D & C.

Making a 'Differential Diagnosis'

Before concluding this chapter it's worth explaining two other disorders which can mimic fibroids, so making what is called a 'differential diagnosis' necessary.

Adenomyosis is a form of endometriosis which can occur within the wall of the womb, where it may be mistaken for fibroids. Endometriosis is the disorder where fragments of the womb lining (the endometrium) are present outside the womb. They are usually to be found on the organs in the pelvis. These fragments respond to the hormonal changes of the menstrual cycle by swelling and bleeding during periods. The result is painful inflammation and the formation of scar tissue around the affected areas. The causes of adenomyosis and endometriosis are unclear.

Both can occur together with fibroids (the woman being childless is the common factor). This may be why some specialists say they encounter fibroids which are not contained tidily in a capsule, but which feed out into the surrounding tissue in a non-cancerous way. Adenomyosis does this and so is more difficult to remove surgically from the womb than fibroids.

More often, though, adenomyosis is a separate problem to fibroids; it may be present in patches or diffused throughout the womb. Like endometriosis, adenomyosis grows in response to the hormones of the menstrual cycle, the womb can become bulky and periods heavy – both of which often indicate fibroids. There may also be pain, which is less usual with fibroids.

Modern trans-vaginal ultrasound is a way of making a differential diagnosis. It can give clues by showing the characteristic spotty 'salt and pepper' appearance of adenomyosis, which is unlike the typical whorling band pattern of fibroids.

The usual treatment is by the same drugs used to shrink endometriosis, such as danazol, buserelin and goserelin. These drugs can also be used to shrink fibroids before surgery to remove them, and we explain how they work on p 53. But if the woman has pelvic pain and a bulky womb, and there is still some uncertainty about the cause, it may be necessary to take a look inside the pelvis to see if endometriosis is present. If there are patches to be seen outside the womb in the pelvis, then this also indicates the likelihood of adenomyosis within the wall of the womb.

Laparoscopy is the procedure used to take a look. It is done under general anaesthetic and is a minor procedure requiring only an overnight stay in hospital. First, harmless carbon dioxide gas is pumped into the abdomen via a fine needle. This inflates the abdomen and separates the pelvic organs, making them easier to see. The patient is tilted slightly head-down, which also helps to separate the intestines from the pelvic organs. A viewing instrument with a light at the end, called a laparoscope, is then inserted through a small incision just inside or below the navel. The laparoscope is no wider than 1 cm (½ in). Endometriosis can be removed during a laparoscopy, if necessary, by minor surgery carried out via another tiny incision just above the pubic hairline.

After a laparoscopy, there may be feelings of heaviness and discomfort in the abdomen, due to the gas. Sometimes there is also pain in the shoulders, known as 'referred pain' because it is referred there from the abdomen by nerves which connect with the diaphragm. Once the gas has been absorbed by the body, usually within a couple of days, these problems disappear and you are rapidly back to normal.

Sometimes more major surgery is needed for both endometriosis and adenomyosis, although drug treatment alone may be effective.

The other condition which can be mistaken for fibroids – and in which stress might play a part - is called **pelvic congestion syndrome**. It is associated with pre-menstrual syndrome (also called pre-menstrual tension or PMT). PMT is a combination of physical and psychological symptoms which occur in the second half of the menstrual cycle, between ovulation and a period. They can include fatigue, irritability, depression, tender breasts, bloated feelings, headache and backache. Pelvic congestion refers to the womb becoming congested with blood at this time, which causes it to enlarge and periods to become heavy; both can mimic fibroids, as we have said before.

Not all women have PMT - or pelvic congestion syndrome with it - but a great many do have some of the symptoms, especially towards the end of their fertile lives; in a few they may be severe. The causes are another uncertainty. A hormone imbalance, in particular a lack of progesterone, may be involved; there may be a deficiency in certain vitamins, such as vitamin B6 and E. It's unclear whether these physical changes cause the stress and tension of PMT, or whether being stressed and anxious for other reasons contributes to it.

However, a woman who was having heavy periods, and who was found to have an enlarged womb when examined by a doctor, would be given an ultrasound scan as a means of making the differential diagnosis. This would show if fibroids or pelvic congestion syndrome were responsible. If pelvic congestion syndrome were diagnosed, then hormone treatment with progestogen (synthetic progesterone) or the pill, plus relaxation techniques and a balanced diet, may help to relieve the syndrome. Chapter 9 on Self-Help would therefore be useful to women with this problem too.

CHAPTER FIVE
Treatments

How fibroids are treated will depend not only on their type and size. The woman's age, her desire to have children, or simply her wish to retain her fertility must be considered. If you are facing treatment for fibroids, there may be a choice and so it is useful to know the options available. This will help you and your gynaecologist to discuss the possible treatments and to decide which is best for you.

If you are in a relationship, it may also be helpful to involve your partner, especially if a proposed treatment would end your fertility, because this is a decision which could affect him too. And if you, or your partner, have any doubts about a treatment which cannot be resolved with your gynaecologist, you can ask your doctor to refer you to another specialist for a second opinion. (You can also ask for further opinions, if you consider it necessary.)

You are not obliged to have any treatment at all (not everyone is aware of this right), but you do need to think carefully about the reasons why it is advisable. Some women, however, are happy to be guided entirely by their gynaecologist, in which case it is still helpful and reassuring to know what to expect. The evidence is that the better informed most patients are, the better they are able to cope with treatments of all kinds.

Hormone treatment, which means taking the pill or progestogen (synthetic progesterone) tablets, may be all that is needed to control heavy periods due to fibroids which aren't causing any other problems. This would continue for six months. If a woman is likely to be starting the menopause (it usually occurs between the ages of 45 and 55), hormone treatment may tide her over until then, when fibroids tend to shrink anyway. This can make surgery unnecessary, but hormones don't always work.

Surgery is the most usual treatment for problem fibroids and there are several ways of carrying it out.

If problems are being caused by small submucous fibroids under the endometrium, or which protrude into the womb cavity, they could be treated by recently developed techniques using the hysteroscope. These techniques can give a woman the choice between keeping her fertility and ending it, without having to undergo major surgery. Called endometrial ablation and endometrial resection, they can be used in two ways:

1 to reduce the size of the fibroids so that periods are returned to normal and fertility is preserved, or

2 to remove the entire womb lining permanently so that periods and fertility are ended.

For either procedure you would be in hospital for no more than a day. Here is what happens, depending on which treatment you have. The procedure would most likely be carried out under a general anaesthetic (see p 65). However, some gynaecologists may give a local anaesthetic by injection into the cervix, plus a sedative, in which case you may be aware of what is happening, though you wouldn't feel any pain. Some women don't remember anything.

After the vaginal area has been thoroughly cleaned with non-stinging antiseptic (although the inside of the vagina cannot be completely sterilized), the cervix is dilated slightly using metal or plastic rods to allow the hysteroscope to be inserted into the womb. Fluid is then run in and out of the womb via a channel in the hysteroscope to keep the view clear during surgery. How the procedure is carried out depends on the gynaecologist's technique and the hospital's equipment, but either of the following could be performed.

1. **Endometrial ablation** uses a powerful beam of laser light for cutting. This is directed into the womb via another channel in the hysteroscope. It can be used to incise individual fibroids away in slivers, and to remove any pedunculated fibroids by severing their stalks, which preserves fertility. Or it can burn

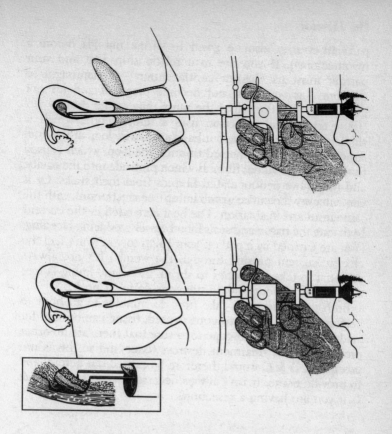

*Small fibroids which protrude into the cavity
of the womb can be removed simply by
resectoscope (above) or by laser, preserving
fertility. Alternatively, the entire womb lining
can be removed by endometrial resection
(below) or by ablation using a laser, which
treats heavy periods and ends fertility.*

the entire womb lining away, permanently ending periods and
fertility. The laser seals tissue at the same time, so reducing
bleeding. Before this treatment you may be given a hormone
drug for about two months to shrink the womb lining so it is
thinner and easier to ablate. Your periods may cease while you
are on it. Drugs which may be used are described later on

p 53 (they may also be given to shrink fibroids before a myomectomy). If you are in a relationship, you and your partner must use barrier contraception - a diaphragm or condom - as you must not become pregnant and it's not possible to take the pill at the same time as the drug.

2. **Endometrial resection** uses a resectoscope, which is similar to a hysteroscope, but has a small wire loop at the end. An electric current is passed through the loop, which is used to shave off individual fibroids which protrude into the cavity, and to remove pedunculated fibroids from their stalks. Or it can cut away the entire womb lining (see illustration), with the same results as in ablation. The heat generated by the current both cuts the tissue and seals blood vessels, reducing bleeding. (You are earthed by a pad on your thigh so you won't feel the electric current passing through the womb.) It's not always essential to take hormones to shrink the womb lining before a resection, although some surgeons do insist on it.

Both procedures can take from 15 minutes to an hour to perform. When a resectoscope is used, tissue can be sent for analysis under a microscope to ensure that there are no other problems. Laser treatment destroys tissue and so this is not possible: a D & C would therefore be carried out beforehand to provide tissue. It isn't always necessary to perform a D & C if you are having a resection.

After either of these procedures, you will spend several hours resting in the recovery room until the sedative or anaesthetic wears off, your blood pressure will be checked, and then you can go home. Arrange for someone to take you because you may be feeling shaky, although this is more of a psychological than a physical reaction. You certainly should not drive.

You will be given painkillers to take if necessary, but you should not be in any severe discomfort. Take things easy for about a week, although many women feel fine after a day or two. It is safe to have a bath or shower the next day.

You may experience slight bleeding and have a blood-stained watery discharge for between one and six weeks, which is normal. If the discharge develops an offensive odour, this can mean you have an infection. If this occurs it is because the vagina is never a sterile environment, not because of any medical negligence. Your doctor can prescribe antibiotics which will clear it. You should use sanitary towels until any discharge ceases, not tampons because they encourage infection. Don't have sex while the discharge lasts. You'll have a formal check-up with your surgeon after about six weeks just to ensure that there are no problems.

Periods usually cease in about 90 per cent of women who have their entire womb lining removed, or there is only slight bleeding at period time. When you resume intercourse following this treatment, continue to use contraception. Even though it is extremely unlikely that you would become pregnant, it is still advisable to take precautions, just in case, until your doctor considers it is no longer necessary. After treatment of fibroids only, your periods should be normal and you could of course become pregnant if you do not use contraception.

Endometrial ablation or resection can only be used to treat small submucous fibroids under the endometrium, or which protrude into the cavity. Larger submucous ones, and troublesome fibroids in other sites, are treated by an abdominal operation. To recap briefly, these fibroids most commonly occur within the muscular wall of the womb, or grow out from it into the abdomen. (Chapter 1 fully describes the sites of fibroids.) The operation to treat them would be either a myomectomy or a hysterectomy. These are both major procedures which merit a separate chapter.

CHAPTER SIX

Myomectomy and Hysterectomy

Because both myomectomy and hysterectomy are major operations, you must feel sure that the right decision is made if either of these procedures would resolve your problem. Myomectomy means removal of fibroids only (myoma = fibroid; ectomy = removal of). In this operation the womb is surgically restored to normal, but there is a risk of fibroids recurring. Hysterectomy means removal of the entire womb ('hystera' or 'hustera' being the Greek word for womb). This operation permanently ends the problem and also the ability to have children.

Women's Feelings

Women often do not realize how they feel about their womb until faced with the possibility of having it removed. Some women aren't concerned about losing it, perhaps because they don't want children, or have all the children they want. Or debilitating problems caused by fibroids may have made having a womb seem just a liability.

Other women can feel quite differently, however. They may still want to have children, or simply wish to retain their womb, perhaps to keep their childbearing options open. For some women, the womb can be a powerful symbol of femininity. A woman can value it as an important part of herself, irrespective of its reproductive role. Its removal could result in a deep sense of loss.

Whatever your feelings, your gynaecologist should take them into consideration when discussing your treatment.

Of course, it is not only your feelings which may count if you have a partner. As we said in the previous chapter, your partner may wish to be involved in a decision about your fertility. In any event, his support and understanding can be most valuable before and after a myomectomy or a hysterectomy, and will be helpful to your relationship after surgery.

You may both be anxious about whether there will be any long-term effects from either operation and how your sex life will be affected (there is more on these aspects later; see chapter 7). Visit your gynaecologist together and discuss any such worries. It may also help your partner to read this book. You will both cope much better the more you can communicate.

Not all men, however, can relate to 'female problems', or you may not be in a relationship with a man. Talking to other women can be most helpful, particularly if you are considering having a hysterectomy. There may be a hysterectomy support group in your area where you can talk to women who have had this operation (but do still rely on your doctor and gynaecologist for medical advice). Your doctor or hospital may be able to put you in touch with a support group; see also Useful Addresses at the end of this book. Each woman's experience of hysterectomy is different, even when it has been carried out for the same problem, so it may be helpful to have several accounts. There are books on hysterectomy listed under Further Reading.

Hysterectomy can be a treatment for cancer. Women who have the operation for this reason have the additional deep anxiety about the disease itself. A support group is likely to include cancer patients and you may well find that their understanding of others' fears is actually all the greater.

There are no myomectomy support groups. Perhaps there should be. You could start one if you decide to have this operation and if talking to other women who have had myomectomies would help. Despite the trauma of facing this major operation, the final result is that the womb is preserved and restored to its normal function. This in itself can be a source of reassurance.

Making the Right Decision

In most cases, there can be a straightforward choice between the two operations. But a myomectomy can sometimes be a longer and more difficult operation than a hysterectomy, depending on the size, position and number of fibroids. Each fibroid has to be 'shelled out' from its capsule and the womb reconstructed, which can require greater skill on the part of the gynaecologist than simply removing the whole womb. This is certainly not a reason against requesting a myomectomy, if that is your preferred option. But if the womb is very misshapen, so that restoring it to normal could be extremely difficult, and the operation might cause excessive bleeding, the gynaecologist will want to reserve the right to carry out a hysterectomy if necessary. This is simply a safeguard. Your permission for this will be asked before the operation, and the surgeon is obliged to discuss it with you. However, it is usually possible to carry out a myomectomy and so the need for a hysterectomy seldom arises.

Understanding Your Operation

Fibroids rarely require emergency treatment and so you are likely to have waiting time before the operation. Knowing what a myomectomy or hysterectomy is likely to involve will help you to prepare for it physically and mentally.

A myomectomy is carried out via an abdominal incision; a hysterectomy is often done this way too. The incision is usually made along the top of the pubic hairline above the womb (a bikini incision), as illustrated. You will probably worry that you will be left with a large scar, but neither a myomectomy nor a hysterectomy leave extensive scarring. Following surgery, the incision heals as a thin red line, but will fade in time to a scarcely noticeable white line, which will be mainly hidden by pubic hair. You will therefore be able to wear a bikini without the scar showing.

Very large fibroids may occasionally necessitate a different incision running vertically up the abdomen from the pubic hairline to somewhere below the navel (a midline incision); the surgeon will endeavour to keep it to the minimum length. This

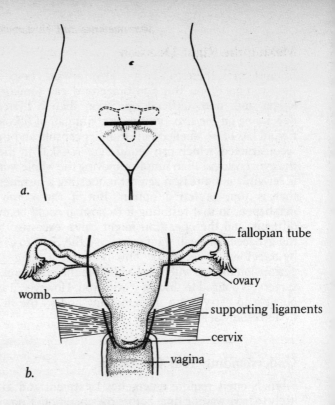

_a._

fallopian tube

ovary

womb

supporting ligaments

cervix

vagina

_b._

a. Usual position of incision for a
   myomectomy or a 'total' abdominal
   hysterectomy for fibroids. The scar will fade
   until it is scarcely noticeable.
b. In a 'total hysterectomy' for fibroids the
   womb and cervix can be removed through
   the abdomen or vagina. The ovaries and
   fallopian tubes are usually left in place.

will also fade to a white line, which will be slightly more
noticeable due to its position. Fortunately, now that one-piece
swimwear is fashionable, you don't have to worry about it
showing when you're on the beach or by the pool.

There may be a further option: if fibroids are small, so that
the womb is enlarged very little, a vaginal hysterectomy could
be carried out. In this operation, the womb is removed from

below, through the vagina rather than through the abdomen, and this leaves no visible scarring.

However, new laparoscopic techniques using a laser or electrodiathermy (a wire heated by electric current) for cutting are becoming available which only involve small abdominal incisions for both myomectomy and hysterectomy. And it is now also possible to remove a bulky womb through the vagina. There is more about these techniques in chapter 8 on New Developments.

Myomectomy

As has already been said, in a myomectomy only the fibroids are taken away, and the womb itself left. For two or three months leading up to the operation you may be recommended to have drug treatment to shrink your fibroids, if they are large. This will make removing them and reconstructing the womb easier. (These drugs may also be used prior to endometrial ablation or resection; see p 44.) Danazol is a drug which may be given. It is most often used to shrink endometriosis, but also has the same effect on fibroids. Taken every day in tablet form, it acts mainly on the pituitary gland and tricks the body into a fake menopause by suppressing the release of FSH and LH; these hormones cause the menstrual cycle to progress. Without them, production of the ovarian hormones oestrogen and progesterone ceases, or is much reduced, depending on the dose. The lack of oestrogen shrinks the fibroids.

It does have adverse side-effects, however, but their severity may vary from woman to woman. They can include hot flushes/flashes, night sweats and other common menopausal symptoms, such as vaginal dryness, loss of libido (sexual desire), fatigue, headaches and mood swings. If danazol is taken for a much longer time, there is the possibility of the voice deepening slightly and some growth of facial hair; this is because it has properties similar to androgens (male hormones). These effects would be extremely unlikely to occur during the short time it was given to shrink fibroids, and are rare anyway even when the drug is used in the longer term. We mention them because women who have heard about danazol sometimes worry unnecessarily about taking the drug.

Any menopausal side-effects which do occur are reversible when it is discontinued.

Increasingly, newer drugs are being used to shrink fibroids because they are more effective. These are called GnRH or LHRH analogues or agonists. GnRH stands for gonadotrophin releasing hormone. Gonadotrophin is a hormone which is responsible for the release of the two pituitary hormones FSH and LH. LHRH stands for luteinizing hormone releasing hormone and is simply another way of describing the same thing. GnRH (or LHRH) analogues are similar in structure to the natural gonadotrophin hormone, but in contrast to it they act mainly on the hypothalamus in the brain to prevent the release of FSH and LH from the pituitary (which is controlled by the hypothalamus). This, again, stops the menstrual cycle, which produces an artificial menopause. Without oestrogen, the fibroids shrink.

The drugs buserelin and goserelin are GnRH/LHRH analogues. They can be given as a nasal spray, as an implant inserted just under the skin of the abdomen, or by daily injection. You can inject yourself, although if you prefer it, a nurse or health care professional at your local health centre can do it.

With both danazol and the analogue drugs, your periods will probably cease and you may become infertile while taking them. But if you have a partner, you and he should still use barrier contraception (a diaphragm or condom) to be on the safe side, as you must not become pregnant while on them, and you cannot take the pill at the same time. The analogues may cause some bone loss (osteoporosis), which happens at the natural menopause, but this is reversible, along with any other menopausal symptoms, when treatment is discontinued. Relaxation techniques, a healthy lifestyle (see Self-Help, chapter 9) and your partner being understanding, if you are in a relationship, will help while any menopausal symptoms last.

This treatment could not be used on its own in the longer term because of the side-effects, and because the fibroids could regrow once it was discontinued.

The Operation

What actually happens during a myomectomy? It is used principally to remove intramural fibroids from the wall of the womb. The surgeon locates the whitish lumps which are fibroids and, using a scalpel, incises into the womb, through the capsule which surrounds a fibroid - avoiding cutting into the fibroid itself - so bleeding is kept to a minimum. By inserting the handle of the scalpel into the capsule, the surgeon can lift out the fibroid (the 'shelling out' referred to earlier). If possible, the surgeon then 'tunnels' from the capsule of the fibroid just removed into the capsule surrounding a nearby fibroid, and 'shells out' that fibroid through the tunnel. This can avoid making other incisions into the womb. More incisions may have to be made, though, and if these are well-placed they may actually weaken the wall less than tunnelling around through one incision.

Some surgeons may operate by laser or electrodiathermy, using them in the manner of a scalpel. These both cut and seal tissue, so reducing bleeding and the risks of infection. The method used will depend on the surgeon's technique and the hospital's equipment. Excellent results can be achieved by a skilful surgeon, whichever method is used.

Although a myomectomy can cause more bleeding than a hysterectomy, excessive bleeding is seldom a serious problem. Drugs which constrict the blood vessels can be injected into the fibroid sites to reduce bleeding if necessary. Even simpler, the uterine arteries bringing blood to the womb can be compressed for a short time to reduce bleeding.

After fibroids have been excised, the empty capsules are closed using soluble stitches, which simply dissolve away inside you during healing. If a bulky womb has stretched the round ligaments which support it, a stitch can be inserted to tighten them up, but this is very seldom needed.

In order to remove cervical fibroids, the bladder has to be pushed forward, away from the womb; its normal position is lying against the cervix and, when pushed, it simply slides off, so the cervix is accessible. The fibroids are then removed, as just described, and the cervix reconstituted.

Pedunculated fibroids, which grow out on a stalk into the

abdomen, are removed by clamping the stalk to cut off the blood supply to the fibroid, tying it with soluble thread (which dissolves away inside you), and then cutting off the fibroid. Similarly, a 'parasitic' fibroid (extremely rare), attached to another organ in the pelvis, will have its blood supply clamped and will then be cut off.

We have already described how submucous fibroids, which grow under the endometrium or out into the cavity of the womb, are removed by laser or resectoscope (see chapter 5). They can also be removed by myomectomy when they occur together with other troublesome fibroids needing this operation.

Hysterectomy

There are several ways of performing a hysterectomy, but the procedure usually used for fibroids is called a 'total hysterectomy'. This operation removes the womb and cervix, which is why it is called 'total'. Originally, surgeons used to leave the cervix (in a 'subtotal hysterectomy'), but this is no longer done because the cervix would remain a potential site for cancer.

In a total abdominal hysterectomy, the womb is freed from its supporting ligaments and blood vessels, which are first clamped, then cut and tied off. The fallopian tubes and the ligaments attaching the ovaries to the womb are also severed. The cervix is detached by making an incision in the top of the vagina, and the entire womb is then lifted out through the opening made in the abdomen. In a total vaginal hysterectomy, the surgeon works from below (which requires more skill), carrying out the procedure through an incision in the top of the vagina, through which the whole womb is removed. A scalpel, laser, or electrodiathermy may be used to carry out these procedures.

You may be wondering how the ovaries and tubes stay in place when no longer attached to the womb, what happens to the space in the pelvis left by the womb, and if there is a hole at the top of the vagina where the cervix once was. The ovaries and tubes do not wander around in an empty space. They are also naturally attached to supporting tissue lining the side walls of the pelvis, which gives them their blood supply, and they remain in this position. There is no hole left at the top of the vagina because it is stitched together. The stitches dissolve during healing (soluble ones are used) leaving a neat scar. To tighten things up, surgeons usually bring across the supporting ligaments and tie them into the top of the vagina when stitching it together. The intestines settle without problems into the space left by the womb.

Removal of the Ovaries

Fibroids in themselves do not necessitate removal of the ovaries during an abdominal hysterectomy (they can't be taken out vaginally, except by the new technique, see p 99). Some surgeons, however, may still want to take them out, particularly if the woman is of an age when the menopause could start. 45, or even 40, is seen by some as - literally - a cut-off age for the ovaries. The reason given for doing this is that it protects the woman against any possibility of developing ovarian cancer. It is not one of the most common cancers, but it tends to occur in women over the age of 40. Against this is the view now held by many surgeons that if the woman is still having regular periods, removing her ovaries with their supply of hormones could have drastic effects.

The ovaries produce the hormones oestrogen and progesterone, upon which the menstrual cycle depends. It is the natural decline in oestrogen at the menopause which causes periods to become irregular and cease; it is also responsible for the other menopausal symptoms already mentioned. In addition, the lack of this hormone leads to the thinning of the bones (osteoporosis). This increases the risks of fractures later in life and causes the round-shouldered look seen in some elderly women, due to bone loss from the spine.

If both ovaries are surgically removed before the menopause, the sudden loss of hormones can cause an artificial menopause which may be more severe than a natural one. Losing their ovaries could also be traumatic for some women; like the womb, they may be valued as part of being female. Although the hormones can be replaced by having HRT (hormone replacement therapy), which can be very effective, it doesn't entirely imitate nature.

It is true that ovarian cancer is usually 'silent' (symptomless) in its early stages and so by the time a woman becomes aware that something is wrong, cancer is often advanced and more difficult to treat. But early screening by ultrasound has improved diagnosis very considerably in recent years. It should therefore be unnecessary to remove the ovaries from most pre-menopausal women to protect them against the relatively small risk of developing ovarian cancer.

We say 'most' because there are exceptions. Women with a family history of ovarian cancer should always tell their doctor and gynaecologist about it (if they don't already know) because, in these women, the risk is considerably increased. This affects women with one or more first-degree relatives (sister, mother or grandmother) who have had ovarian cancer. These women must be screened regularly, and in their case it is worth removing the ovaries as a preventive measure when the opportunity arises, such as during a hysterectomy for fibroids. (There is also something to be said in favour of removing the ovaries from a woman without this risk if they are failing naturally and there are increasing gaps between periods.) But provided that other pre-menopausal women have regular check-ups, they will be adequately protected.

Even though many surgeons today would leave the ovaries in a pre-menopausal woman with no family history of ovarian cancer, it is still worthwhile ensuring that you understand exactly what will be done during a hysterectomy for fibroids before consenting to it.

Being Constructive

There are several constructive ways in which you can use the time before admission to hospital for a myomectomy or hysterectomy. You will cope far better with the operation if you improve your general health – and this includes your morale – as much as possible.

A balanced diet and taking exercise will obviously contribute to your physical well-being and this can have direct benefits where your operation is concerned.

If you are in good shape, you will heal better than if you are overweight. A woman who is very overweight may well be asked to lose weight before the operation. This is because there are technical difficulties in performing abdominal operations on the overweight; healing also takes longer and the risks of infection are greater. In some cases, the gynaecologist may be reluctant to operate because of the risks. If your doctor or gynaecologist advises you to lose weight, it is certainly sensible to try and do so. In addition, if you can maintain the right weight for your size, the chances of large fibroids recurring after a myomectomy may be reduced. This doesn't mean you have to conform to a fashionable stereotype of slimness, but excessive weight can be a health hazard in many ways, so being the weight advised by your doctor also has other long-term advantages.

Giving up smoking, or cutting down at least, if you are a smoker, is very important too. This is not only because of the well-known risks associated with smoking, but because of particular risks after surgery. Smokers produce more mucus in the bronchial tubes of their lungs, and they are therefore more liable to chest problems and pneumonia after a general anaesthetic. Patients are reluctant to cough, particularly following an abdominal operation, as it hurts and can disrupt the stitches. So the mucus is not removed and this encourages infection. Smoking isn't permitted in a hospital ward anyway, not simply because of the risks to the smoker, but because 'passive smoking' (inhaling someone else's smoke) is a danger to the health of other patients and staff. You would have to go into the day room, or be in a private room, if you want to smoke. Those who are able to give up smoking in preparation for an operation often find they have managed to quit for good – and so their health also benefits in the longer term.

As has already been mentioned, it is not simply your physical health which matters, however. Improving your morale is also important. The prospect of having a major operation is stressful for virtually everyone, which is only to be expected. But if you are calm and relaxed you may have less pain and recover faster. This is where alternative therapies can be especially helpful when used together with orthodox medical treatment. Chapter 9 on Self-Help, gives you advice on alternative (or complementary) therapies and on ways of improving your general health.

Getting Organized

For a myomectomy or hysterectomy you will be in hospital for about a week, and you should allow about a month to recover afterwards. Use the time before going into hospital to organize the practical side of your life too, so you won't be worrying about things at home or at work while you are in hospital and during recovery.

- Stock up the freezer, especially if you have a family to feed.

- Give your home a thorough clean and tidy, so you won't be anxious about coming home to a muddle.

- If you live alone, remember to cancel delivery of milk and newspapers - and lock up your home securely when you go into hospital. It's also wise to arrange for someone to keep an eye on your home in your absence and to do such things as watering plants.

- Make arrangements for the care of any family members and pets. You may need a home help, though this depends on how much a partner, relatives or friends can do while you are in hospital and during recovery. Your doctor, or the hospital social worker, may be able to put you in touch with local services which provide domestic help.

- If you go out to work, ensure that your employer is fully informed about your situation and that you can claim any sickness benefits due to you.

- Arrange for transport to the hospital and home again after the operation. The hospital may be able to help with this if necessary. Try to have someone with you - a partner, relative or friend - especially when you leave the hospital.

- Consider the question of visitors. Immediately after the operation you won't be feeling good and are very unlikely to want any visitors until a day or two later, except perhaps for someone close to you. You could arrange beforehand for one person to let the others know how you are and when you feel up to seeing them. In a hospital ward, you may not be allowed more than two visitors at a time, to minimize disturbance. Voluntary workers and ministers of religion make regular visits to hospitals. They are sensitive to patients' feelings and won't pressure you to talk if you don't feel like it. But don't hesitate to make your wishes clear, if you need to. However, visitors, flowers and 'get well' cards are all good for the morale, so don't deter people unless you really feel you must.

Going Into Hospital

You will receive a letter of admission from the hospital which will give you the date and time to arrive, and tell you where to go in the hospital. You may also be sent information about the hospital and advice on preparing for surgery. Here are some general guidelines which are appropriate to a myomectomy or hysterectomy.

● As for all gynaecological procedures, you must not be having a period at the time of surgery, so check when yours is due and notify the hospital if the date is unsuitable.

● If you are taking the combined oestrogen/progestogen contraceptive pill, you will need to come off it about a month before the operation because oestrogen encourages blood clots to form after major surgery. Use a barrier method of contraception, such as a diaphragm or condom. It is safe to continue taking the progestogen-only pill, although of course you will not need contraception any more if you are having a hysterectomy. But if you are taking a drug to shrink your fibroids, you will need to use a barrier method, as you cannot be on the pill at the same time.

● Notify the hospital if you have any other ailment, such as a cold, when you are due to be admitted, because this might make the operation inadvisable. A heavy cold may affect your breathing under a general anaesthetic.

Things to Take With You

When deciding on the things you will need to take into hospital, imagine that you're going to stay in a hotel (though you won't need many clothes).

- Take nightwear, washing things and other items you may use regularly, such as moisturiser, hand cream, paper tissues, talc and a cologne stick or spray.
- Reading can help pass the time before and after the operation, so you may want to take in some books and magazines.
- If you intend to write letters or cards, take a pen, stationery and stamps.
- You may be able to buy most of the above from the hospital shops or ward trolley when it comes round, so have a little money with you.
- You may also need some change for making phone calls, although in a private room there will be a telephone by the bed and any calls will be charged to your account.
- Being in hospital is a good opportunity to do such things as knitting, sewing, crochet or embroidery, if you enjoy them, and they will help pass the time too.
- You can take in a radio (if it has an earpiece or headphones), although the hospital may provide one. Some hospitals have their own radio station. Programmes may include putting patients in touch with each other via chat shows and playing their special music requests.
- You could also take in a cassette player with headphones so you can listen to your favourite tapes.
- If you have a very small portable TV you may be allowed to use it in a ward, if it has headphones. There will be a TV in the day room; in a private room, radio and TV are provided.
- Don't take in any valuables, such as jewellery or a watch (unless it's plastic).

● Photos of loved ones, and even that old cuddly toy, will cheer you up (plenty of people take in a much-loved mascot, so there's nothing silly about doing this, if you want to).

In Hospital

When you arrive, admission forms need to be filled in and you'll be given an identity bracelet to wear. Don't take this off before you leave hospital.

Once you are in your ward or room, you may be asked to undress straight away and put on your dressing gown. A doctor will examine you and make routine checks, such as your blood pressure, heart and lungs; this is easier if you are undressed. A blood sample will also be taken. It is tested to determine your blood group, so that it can be matched with donor blood, just in case you need a transfusion after surgery. All blood donated for transfusions is screened for hepatitis and HIV (the virus associated with causing AIDS), so there is no longer a risk of infection.

To ensure that the operation will be safe for you, the doctor will ask about your medical history, whether you are currently taking any medicines, and whether you have any allergies. You will be requested to hand over any medicines you have and these will be given to you as required.

You will already have discussed your operation with your own doctor and gynaecologist. Even so, the hospital doctor will also want to discuss it with you. This is to ensure that you really do understand what will be done and are in agreement with it. If you are unclear about anything, this is the time to be absolutely certain your questions are answered. Write them down beforehand, so you can't forget what you wanted to ask. Use the space provided at the end of this book for Notes and Questions, and take the book into hospital with you. Your surgeon (who may be your consultant gynaecologist, or one of his/her senior staff) and the anaesthetist may also visit you. Take these opportunities to ask questions, if necessary.

As with all operations to be carried out under general anaesthetic, whether major or minor, your written consent is needed. This means signing a consent form. Read it carefully and thoroughly. If there is anything you're not sure about, don't hesitate to ask for an explanation. It is your right, and the hospital has a duty to explain the form. You are not obliged to sign it, if you don't want to; your treatment can always be reconsidered, even at this late stage, if this is what you want. Having treatment is entirely voluntary and you can leave hospital whenever you wish.

If it is your first major operation, you are likely to find it all somewhat nerve-racking, which is quite normal. Even if you've had hospital treatment before, and so have a better idea of what to expect, you may still feel anxious. But when any fears you may have about treatment are resolved, you will probably feel much more positive: fear and anxiety are often caused by uncertainty. Doctors and nurses are sometimes criticized for not being sufficiently good communicators, but they cannot always know what is on your mind. Reading this book, and having it with you in hospital, will help you to decide what you need to ask.

It is worth adding that if you are in a teaching hospital, the consultant may visit you with a small group of medical students. They will want to discuss your case, ask you questions and perhaps examine you, as part of their training. You are under no obligation to agree to this, but if you feel you can participate, you will have helped to educate a new generation of doctors. You might also be asked to take part in a research project. If so, what is involved must be fully explained to you, as must any effects it might have on you. Similarly, the decision to participate is entirely yours.

Before the Operation

If your operation is scheduled for the morning, you'll be admitted to hospital the day before; if it's in the afternoon or evening, you'll be admitted the same morning or early afternoon. You won't be given anything to eat for at least four hours prior to the operation, so there will be no risk of your being sick and inhaling vomit under the anaesthetic. This rule about eating applies to any procedure carried out under general anaesthetic, or which might necessitate one.

The time before the operation will pass more quickly and

easily if you occupy yourself in the ways already suggested. Or you may simply wish to relax, meditate, think or pray. For many people, however, one of the most rewarding aspects of being in hospital is getting to know other patients. They can often be most supportive, encouraging and helpful to each other.

Preparations for the operation start about two hours before. Prior to a myomectomy or hysterectomy, your pubic hair needs to be removed, either by shaving or a depilatory cream (the hospital will provide these). A nurse can do it for you, although you will probably prefer to do it yourself, before you take a bath or shower. Removing pubic hair can make some women feel vulnerable, perhaps because it changes their intimate appearance back to an almost childlike state, but it does regrow quite fast and helps to hide the scar.

Put on the theatre gown and cap provided (the opening in the gown goes at the back). Contact lenses or dentures must be removed. No make-up, nail polish or jewellery can be worn, although a special ring you may want to keep on can be taped over.

These final preparations can be very unnerving and this is the time when you are most likely to feel physical fear of pain and even death. The truth is that you won't feel a thing during the operation. Anaesthetists are highly skilled specialists and the dose of anaesthetic is carefully measured to suit your needs. Afterwards, you will be given painkillers whenever necessary (there is more about pain relief on p 69). The chances of anything going wrong are extremely remote - people very seldom die on the operating table, whatever you may have heard - so you certainly should not worry. It is because problems are so very rare that they make headlines when they happen. You will be the centre of attention during the run-up to surgery and the nurses will reassure you.

About an hour before the operation you will be given a pre-medication injection or tablet. This will make you feel sleepy and relaxed. You will be lifted on to a trolley when it's time for the operation, and a hospital porter will wheel you to the theatre. A nurse will also go with you and may hold your hand, to reassure you; your surgeon may greet you when you arrive, although you probably won't remember much about all this. The anaesthetist will inject anaesthetic into a vein in the back of your hand, after which you won't be aware of anything.

There is a very common minor worry which it is worth commenting on here, since people are often reluctant to ask about it. This is whether they are likely to talk under anaesthetic and perhaps reveal personal details they'd rather others didn't know. The answer is that you can't talk during a major operation because a breathing tube is inserted down your throat, although people sometimes chatter incoherently when 'coming round' afterwards.

Afterwards

When you regain consciousness following a myomectomy or hysterectomy you will, of course, feel drowsy. You may also feel sick and actually be sick. This is also a result of the anaesthetic. It is less usual with modern anaesthetics, but people react in varying ways. If nausea is severe, you can be given an injection to quell it.

Your mouth will be dry and you may feel very thirsty. This is due partly to the pre-medication injection, which dries saliva and urine, and partly to the tube the anaesthetist puts down your throat into your trachea (windpipe) to oxygenate you during the operation. This tube is necessary because the anaesthetist also gives you a muscle relaxant, which enables the surgeon to divide the abdominal muscles (they're not cut through) more easily. The relaxant also affects your other muscles, including those controlling breathing, so the tube helps you to breathe. (A relaxant isn't needed before minor procedures, such as a D & C and hysteroscopy, so breathing is normal.)

Unfortunately, it's not possible to have a drink straight after major surgery. The digestive system tends to shut down, due to the anaesthetic and because of the disturbance to the intestines during surgery (they're packed out of the way with sterile swabs during an abdominal operation). A drink could make you sick; sips of water are allowed, or you may be given a piece of ice to suck.

You will find yourself attached to various tubes. These can look alarming to someone who is unprepared, but they are not a sign that anything is wrong and they are painless.

You'll be on a drip. This replaces fluid lost during surgery and rehydrates you because you can't drink directly afterwards. The fluid in the drip is constituted to be similar to your own body fluids. It is given via a slim tube attached to a needle which is inserted into a vein in the back of your hand or arm; this is taped in position. The tube leads to a bag of fluid attached to a stand by the bed. Pain relief can also be given in the same drip.

It is unlikely that you will need a blood transfusion following a myomectomy or hysterectomy, but occasionally it is necessary to replace blood lost during the operation. This is given in the same way as a drip. As explained earlier, the blood given will have been matched to your own blood group and screened for infection.

You may have a drain. This is a tube inserted through the skin at the side of an abdominal incision; it is held in place by a couple of stitches. The tube passes below the fibrous sheath which underlies the skin (both the skin and the fibrous sheath are cut during surgery). It goes underneath the incision, which has of course been stitched together. Any internal bleeding beneath the incision is thus removed via the tube.

Not all surgeons put in a drain, but many do, and the most usual kind is called a suction drain; this gently sucks out blood and drains it into a bottle under the bed. Some surgeons insert a corrugated rubber drain through the incision and under the fibrous sheath; this doesn't use suction, but allows blood to track along the drain into a bottle or bag under the bed, or into an absorbent pad on the abdomen, which is changed as necessary. Occasionally, a drain going deeper into the pelvis is needed if there has been a lot of bleeding during surgery. This is likely, for instance, if the woman has adhesions (scar tissue) caused by endometriosis or infection, from which the womb has had to be detached. This leaves more raw surface. There may therefore be a couple of tubes from the abdomen. A drain from the incision in the vagina following a hysterectomy is rarely needed, even when the womb has been removed through the vagina.

A catheter - a tube to help you urinate - is seldom required. However, by the time many women are having surgery for fibroids, they have also reached an age when stress incontinence (slight leakage of urine on coughing, sneezing, laughing or sudden exertion) is not uncommon. This is due to a mild prolapse (downward displacement) of the bladder neck, which may have resulted from childbearing or an activity which strains the supporting pelvic floor muscles; it can simply be part of the ageing process. Fibroids are unlikely to be a cause, but they might make the problem worse.

Often the problem is not serious enough to justify a separate operation, and sometimes doing certain exercises which strengthen the supporting muscles can help; see p 79. But if a woman is having a hysterectomy or a myomectomy, it can be combined with a repair to the bladder neck. During a vaginal hysterectomy, a triangle of loose skin can be removed from inside the front vaginal wall. The skin edges, and the firm connective tissue which underlies the skin, are brought together and stitched. This buttresses the bladder neck, lifting it back into position (the procedure is known as a Kelly repair). Soluble stitches are used, which dissolve away. The healed area continues to support the bladder neck. Similarly, during an abdominal hysterectomy or a myomectomy, permanent stitches can be placed each side of the vagina and then attached to the ligaments each side of the pubic bone; these stitches lift the vagina and the neck of the bladder with it. The operation is called colposupension.

If a repair is done, then a catheter is put in straight away (it drains into a bottle or bag under the bed). A catheter may be inserted into the urethra - the passage through which you urinate - or straight into the bladder through the abdominal wall at the pubic hairline; this is called a supra-pubic catheter. It helps to reduce the risk of infection, which is slightly more likely with a urethral catheter. This is not due to any contamination, but because it can cause mild bruising to the urethra and this makes the area susceptible to infection.

A supra-pubic catheter also allows the woman to try to urinate normally while it is in place. Women often worry if they can't urinate right away after a repair, but it is quite usual for it to take a few days. To remove the catheter, the tube is gently pulled out; the bladder and abdominal wall heal naturally afterwards.

A catheter isn't necessary otherwise following a

hysterectomy or myomectomy - unless you have trouble urinating after the operation, which happens just very occasionally. You must urinate within twelve hours of surgery to prevent the bladder from becoming over-distended, which could happen because you are drowsy from the anaesthetic and don't realize it is full. The nurses will ensure that you do pass water and will help you on to a bedpan or commode. It is easiest to use this in a private room; in a ward the curtains will be drawn around your bed, and there is at least the consolation of knowing that other patients have to do it this way too, which can help you to overcome any inhibitions. If necessary, the nurses may encourage you by turning on the taps in your ward or room.

If you can't manage it, a catheter will be inserted. It may be placed in the urethra, which shouldn't hurt if insertion is done carefully, although it may be a little uncomfortable when in place. Or it may be inserted supra-pubically; the skin of the abdomen is frozen by an injection before the tube is put through a small opening made in the abdominal wall.

Any such tubes will be removed within two or three days of the operation. Removal is done by gently pulling them out, which ought not to cause any pain, although removal of a urethral catheter or a drain may sometimes be uncomfortable.

Pain Relief

There is absolutely no need to suffer pain in hospital these days. We all have different levels of sensitivity to pain and you should always say if you are in pain, since it isn't easy for others to gauge how you feel. You may find that the nurses ask you very frequently if you have any pain. But - as was said earlier - if you are in a calm and positive state of mind, you may be less sensitive to pain anyway (see Self-Help, chapter 9).

Pain relief can be given in various ways. For instance, while you are still in the operating theatre under general anaesthetic, the anaesthetist may inject a long-acting local anaesthetic, which infiltrates an abdominal wound and gives relief for up to 36 hours. This is usually long enough for you to be over any severe pain. Meanwhile, the incision will feel numb.

Straight after the operation, pain relief can be given by drip (as previously described), or by injection into your buttock or thigh. It can be taken by mouth in tablet form when your digestive system is working again. Painkillers can make you feel drowsy.

Another method of giving pain relief following a hysterectomy is by epidural. An epidural is an injection into the lower spine which numbs you from the waist down. Its use after hysterectomy is not standard practice, but it is sometimes available. It is also given while you are still in the operating theatre under general anaesthetic. A fine hollow needle is inserted into the epidural space which surrounds the spinal cord, a slim tube is passed down the needle, and the needle is then withdrawn, leaving the tube which is taped in place. Painkillers are injected down the tube at the required rate by syringe pump when you are conscious; this is done by a nurse. You won't feel drowsy with this method of pain relief and the tube can be left in place for two or three days.

An epidural is frequently used in childbirth, but when given for labour pains or a Caesarean birth, it affects your bladder function and ability to move below the waist. This kind doesn't have these side-effects, but it isn't used in childbirth because it wouldn't work as well as it does for post-operative pain.

A further interesting development is the use of acupuncture in hospital. As yet, few hospitals offer this 'alternative' form of pain relief, but it is gaining ground, and can also be used to relieve nausea. Acupuncture involves the insertion of very fine needles into specific points on the body (this is virtually painless); there is more about why it may work on p 109. It could also help you during convalescence at home.

Just as interesting is the recent use in orthodox medicine of the positive power of suggestion. At Glasgow Royal Infirmary, hysterectomy patients are played tapes while under general anaesthetic in the operating theatre; these give messages such as, 'Your operation will be successful, you feel warm and comfortable, any pain will not concern you.' Women who are played these tapes need less post-operative pain-relief than those who aren't.

In case you are concerned that discomfort will keep you awake at night in hospital, it's worth mentioning that sleeping pills will be offered, but you could try the relaxation techniques given in the self-help chapter, to see if they work for you. The nurses will do their best to make you comfortable, and will try to keep disturbance in a ward to a minimum, although the care of patients makes some noise inevitable. Some nurses are trained in aromatherapy (massage with essential oils; see chapter 9). They find that patients who receive this kind of massage sleep better and have less pain than those who do not. Like acupuncture, it is not yet available in many hospitals, but if it is offered in yours, it could be well worth having.

Post-Operative Problems

Post-operative problems affect about half of all women after a hysterectomy. They are rarely serious and can usually be resolved quite easily. As has already been said, the most common risk is of infection, due to the wound at the top of vagina. The vagina can never be a sterile environment because it is open to the air in which bacteria are always present.

Signs of infection are a smelly, discoloured discharge, or heavy vaginal bleeding a few days after the operation. It can be treated successfully with antibiotics; some gynaecologists give them routinely via a drip as a preventive measure. This isn't to say that infection is inevitable.

A heavy loss of blood soon after the operation can be due to a haemorrhage (bleeding from the vaginal wound), rather than infection. This can happen because the skin of the vagina is a relatively thin layer - compared to the abdomen - and so a blood vessel on the edge of the incision may give way. It can be necessary to insert a further stitch under general anaesthetic to stop the bleeding. If this happens you may be in hospital for about a day longer and need a blood transfusion.

It is normal to bleed lightly after either a myomectomy or a hysterectomy, and you will be wearing a sanitary towel. Bleeding after a myomectomy is unlikely to continue for more than a day or two. After a hysterectomy, you will have a bloodstained discharge for a few weeks. Continue to use sanitary towels, as tampons increase the risk of infection.

Infection can be a risk following a myomectomy, but it is not usually as great as after a hysterectomy. There is no wound at the top of the vagina to become infected or cause heavy bleeding. However, there may be more bleeding during the operation, and where there is blood there can also be the risk of infection, so some gynaecologists also give antibiotics routinely by drip afterwards, as has already been mentioned. There can be bleeding inside the wall of the womb where it has been cut to remove fibroids. This can cause the womb to become tense (swollen), but the blood is reabsorbed.

Sometimes a blood clot (a haematoma) can form just under the skin of an abdominal incision following either operation. A drain is not needed to prevent this because it can escape through the wound, if necessary, unlike bleeding beneath the fibrous sheath which underlies the skin; this is why a drain which runs underneath can be needed because a collection of blood there can weaken the wound.

The surgeon would endeavour to tie off or seal (using a heated diathermy probe) blood vessels in the incision, to prevent them from bleeding. But when you are under anaesthetic your blood pressure is low and as you recover consciousness, blood pressure rises, so smaller blood vessels which weren't bleeding before may start leaking. This leakage of blood can collect just under the skin and may feel tender, like a bruise. It may be reabsorbed during healing or be spontaneously discharged through the wound; it may form a small hard lump, which can be released by a doctor or nurse making a small separation in the wound by using tweezers gently. If a haematoma gets infected, it can form a small abscess, called a stitch abscess, but this is not serious and will discharge by itself, or can be released as just described.

A haematoma is quite a common occurrence and women often worry about this release of blood because they think it is coming from deep inside, but it is actually a trivial thing on the surface. Only a dressing is required until it dries up completely after a few days.

The bladder may become susceptible to infection after a hysterectomy because the womb is cut away from it. Any bruising to the area during surgery may also make it liable to infection. Pain or burning on urination are signs of this, but it can also be treated successfully with antibiotics.

Removal of Stitches

An abdominal incision may be covered by a dressing to start with, which will be removed within a couple of days. The incision will then be protected by a fine plastic film which is sprayed on. But not all surgeons use a dressing. Instead, the incision may be protected from the beginning by the plastic spray-on film which will wash off before your stitches are removed.

Some women find it difficult to look at the incision initially, even though all there is to see is a neat, thin red line, stitched together. Looking at it in the mirror may be easier at first because this is somehow more impersonal and enables you to see that it is not disfiguring.

The stitches (known medically as sutures) will be removed by a doctor or nurse in about five to seven days, before you leave hospital. An abdominal incision may be stitched with silk or synthetic thread, and the method used depends on the gynaecologist's technique. For instance, 'interrupted' stitches are inserted individually and so each stitch is cut and removed separately. Or a 'continuous thread' stitch may be used; this is called a sub-cuticular suture because it runs under the surface of the skin and is pulled tight to close the incision. It is secured with a bead and a metal clip at each end, and slips straight out when one end is cut free and the other pulled. Sometimes a row of metal clips closes the incision, and these are also removed individually. Removal of stitches or clips should not hurt if done carefully. Deeper soluble stitches may be inserted in an abdominal incision and these don't need to be removed because they dissolve away.

Soluble sutures are used for internal stitches and for closing the top of the vagina after a hysterectomy. These don't need to be removed either as they simply dissolve away. After a myomectomy you may feel tingling sensations in the abdomen within about two weeks as the soluble stitches in the womb dissolve.

Recovery

You will start recovering from a myomectomy or hysterectomy while you are still in hospital. The doctor or surgeon will check you the day after the operation. Everything being satisfactory - as is usually the case - the nurses will help you to get out of bed and to walk around. You will also be encouraged to sit out of bed during the day.

This may seem very soon after a major operation, but walking around is essential to keep your circulation going and to prevent blood clots from forming in your legs as a result of being immobile in bed. Any tubing, plus bottles or bags attached, can be carried with you, and a nurse will carry the drip stand. Should you be unable to get up for any reason, you will need to do foot exercises or have your legs massaged. Sometimes anti-coagulant drugs are given.

Although you'll be on painkillers, you'll still feel you have to move very carefully. This is just as well if you've had an abdominal operation since it is essential not to put any strain on the incision at this early stage. It's worth knowing a couple of techniques which can make moving on your own easier when you first attempt it.

The nurses will arrange your pillows to support you in bed, but to help yourself sit up and lie down straight after surgery, you could take a strong cord into hospital (such as a man's dressing gown cord) which is long enough to tie to the foot of the bed. You can pull yourself up and lower yourself on this.

When getting out of bed, roll on to one side with your knees bent up, raise yourself on your elbow and swing your legs over the side of the bed, using your arms to push yourself into a sitting position. Simply reverse this sequence when getting back into bed: sit on the edge, lower yourself on your arms and swing your legs up, then roll on to your back.

You won't be able to straighten up right away after an abdominal operation, but don't worry about this. Your posture will improve as you heal. Being 'bent over' may be partly a psychological reaction. A woman who'd had a myomectomy described it as 'perhaps being a self-protective reflex, since it didn't actually hurt me to stand up straight; surgery can leave you feeling vulnerable'. You may also feel fragile and unsteady, and this too can be as much psychological as it is physical. Having a major operation is a shock to the system.

The hospital physiotherapist will visit you and explain exercises you can do to strengthen muscles affected by surgery.

See the section later in this chapter on post-operative exercises. Start them as soon as you feel able.

Make every effort to move around, because it also encourages your digestive system to start working again. You should be able to drink normally the day after the operation and to eat about two days later. You probably won't have much appetite and solid food may not appeal. This isn't necessarily because hospital food is not always as good as it should be - even the most enticing dishes can seem offputting at this stage. Start with something light and smooth, such as ice cream, jelly or creamed potatoes. Prepared 'meals in a drink', which are highly nutritious, may be available in hospital, or can be bought in pharmacies and taken into hospital with you. Do try to eat some solid food as soon as possible.

Because the digestive system has been out of action, it may not function fully right away and wind tends to build up. This can cause discomfort and make your abdomen swell. Not all women have wind, but it is very common, so don't feel embarrassed. When you open your bowels, this should relieve the problem. Some women find it recurs for a while after they've left hospital: 'I had a pot belly for several months after my hysterectomy', is how one woman described it. Drinking soda or peppermint water will help you to bring up wind, and the nurses can provide other remedies.

An important part of recovery is feeling that you are regaining control, and this too can begin in hospital. Simple things like washing yourself and doing your hair will raise your morale, especially if you're expecting visitors. To start with, the nurses will do these things for you, but you should feel brighter within a couple of days of the operation and be able to do them for yourself. You can have a shower after about 24 hours and this will also help you to feel brighter and fresher. Don't rub an abdominal incision; just gently pat it dry. Some hospitals provide hairdressing and manicure services, either on the premises or hired in, and you can take advantage of these. If you look good, you are likely to feel better.

Before you leave hospital, a doctor or your gynaecologist will check you and when you get home you can see your own doctor if necessary. Your gynaecologist will want to check you again after six weeks. These are opportunities to discuss any problems.

Convalescence at Home

Bear in mind that when you first get home you may feel very tired, much more so than you did in hospital, even though you are actually recovering. A hospital provides a supportive environment with an established routine which you are likely to miss. To speed recovery, you could perhaps spend a week or two at a convalescent home, and the hospital may be able to help arrange this. However, recuperation after a myomectomy or hysterectomy for fibroids should be quicker and easier than if you'd had a more extensive abdominal operation, as is sometimes needed for cancer. Recovery from a vaginal hysterectomy for fibroids is quickest of all because there is no abdominal incision nor any disturbance to the underlying muscles.

Many books advising on recovery after hysterectomy describe the 'stages' of convalescence, detailing what you can and cannot do at each stage, up to a period of three months. There is no such advice available for myomectomy because this is the first book devoted entirely to the subject of fibroids.

There is actually very little difference in recovery from either operation, and medical experts are increasingly abandoning the 'three months of convalescence' programme for hysterectomy. The approach is to encourage women to be as active as possible early on, aiming for a complete return to normal life within about a month to six weeks.

This isn't to say that you should feel pressured or inadequate if you can't meet this target. Much depends on your general state of health and fitness before the operation, but it is sensible to try and be in the best possible shape before surgery, as advised earlier in the book. The overall post-op advice is to do as much as you can, but to listen to your body. Don't push yourself too hard, so that you become exhausted, and you certainly should not do anything which causes pain.

Exercises

In the words of Professor Stuart Campbell, 'I would advise early activity, gradually increasing the amount of exercise you do, which means doing as much as you feel capable of. Get

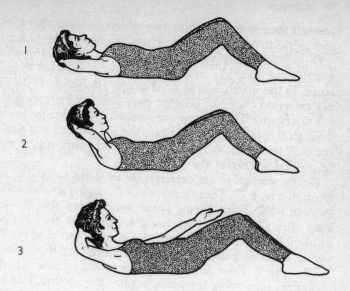

Gentle exercises to firm and strengthen
abdominal muscles following a myomectomy
or hysterectomy. To be carried out daily.

1. Lie on your back, hands behind your head
   and elbows on the floor. Place feet and
   knees parallel, about 30 cm (12 in) apart.
   Breathe in deeply.

2. Lift your head and shoulders off the floor a
   little, using your abdominal muscles, not
   your arms, until you can see your knees.
   Breathe out slowly as you lift and breathe
   in as you lower. Repeat 4 times to start
   with.

3. As before, but reach through your knees
   with one hand, then repeat with the other
   hand. Breathe out as you reach, inhale as
   you release. Repeat 4 times.

As you recover, increase the number of times
you repeat the exercises.

yourself into systematic exercises which improve abdominal and pelvic floor muscle tone. These are of positive benefit.'

During an abdominal hysterectomy or a myomectomy the muscles are divided and stretched (though not cut) to gain access to the womb, and so need toning afterwards. If they're not exercised they can become even flabbier, increasing the risk of a hernia. This is a rupture where the intestine protrudes through the abdominal wall when the muscles are put under stress. A tender lump forms under the skin and surgery may be needed to correct the problem.

Gentle strengthening exercises, to be done every day, are illustrated on p 77. There is no risk of damaging an abdominal incision while doing them. These muscles can also become slack after a vaginal hysterectomy, even though they are not involved in the operation, since the womb is removed via the vagina. Exercising them is still worthwhile to keep them toned.

The pelvic floor muscles run across the base of the abdomen, supporting the pelvic organs: the urethra, bladder, vagina, womb - if it remains - and rectum (see illustration). The muscles are not directly affected by these operations and may positively benefit from surgery: during a hysterectomy the ligaments at the sides which were attached to the womb are usually brought across and tied into the top of the vagina, which tightens up the pelvic floor. Even so, lack of exercise can cause them to lose tone, creating the conditions which may lead later on to a prolapse (downward displacement of any of the pelvic organs). Surprisingly, perhaps, even a womb made bulky by fibroids doesn't weigh down and stretch the pelvic floor very much because its size prevents it from slipping through the pelvis. But, for the reasons just given, it is still worthwhile exercising the pelvic floor muscles after a myomectomy. And if a repair for stress incontinence (leakage of urine) was combined with a hysterectomy or myomectomy, exercise can help to prevent this problem recurring.

There are other advantages too. The pelvic area may lose sensitivity following a hysterectomy, which can have a very negative effect on your sex life. Gynaecological problems and surgery can be a sexual turn-off anyway, but doing pelvic floor exercises will help to resolve any such difficulties. There is advice on restarting intercourse in the next chapter.

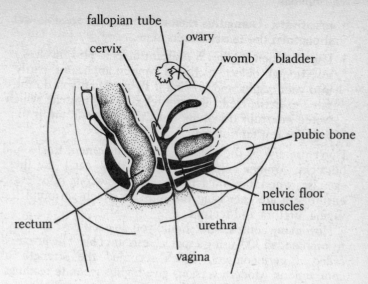

fallopian tube
ovary
cervix
womb   bladder
pubic bone
pelvic floor
muscles
rectum
urethra
vagina

Exercises which strengthen the supporting
pelvic floor muscles are of benefit following
surgery.

These simple pelvic floor exercises were devised some years ago by Dr Arnold Kegel, an American gynaecologist, and so are often called Kegel exercises. He intended them to prevent stress incontinence following childbirth but they are now widely recommended simply to improve muscle tone. Sex manuals include them as a means of improving sexual response and helping women to reach orgasm. They involve being able to do three things.

1 When urinating, contract your pelvic floor muscles to stop the flow of urine and then release them. If you can't do this, your muscles definitely need toning and you should practise by repeating this contraction, as if you were stopping the flow of urine, whenever you remember. You can do it anywhere without people knowing what you are doing.

2 If you can do the first exercise, take it a stage further by holding the contraction to a count of five before

releasing it. Doing this exercise as often as possible will strengthen the muscles even more.

3 Exercise them against a resistant object. This involves inserting an object, such as a tampon applicator, partly into your vagina and holding it there. Then you do the same exercise, clenching and relaxing the muscles which would interrupt urination, but this time your aim is to grip the resistant object.

Don't use any of the muscles in your abdomen, thighs and buttocks. Women sometimes think they can't do these exercises when they are actually using the wrong muscles, so ensure you are exercising the muscles which surround the vagina, urethra and rectum.

How many contractions should you do each day? Dr Kegel recommended 300, using a special resistant object he invented called a perineometer, which recorded the strength of contractions. Modern versions give highly accurate readings, but whether you use one of these, or a tampon applicator, you should soon be able to do the exercises without a resistant object. You can then practise anywhere, without anyone knowing. Don't worry about reaching the 300 target (keeping count could be impossible anyway); being able to do all the exercises described here is what matters.

Exercising your whole body is also important in recovery and in preventing the weight gain which can so often happen after a major operation. We advise on ways of regaining your general fitness on p 105.

Heavy Lifting

Much traditional advice following major abdominal surgery cautions against heavy lifting. The fact is that heavy lifting, if done incorrectly, is bad for anyone, whether or not they've had a major operation.

Professor Campbell again: 'I think we exaggerate about the dangers of heavy lifting. We should counsel more towards exercising abdominal and pelvic floor muscles. If you don't keep the muscles in good tone, you're more likely to get a prolapse or a hernia. We should encourage women to resume normal life, not to avoid lifting and activity.'

This doesn't mean that you should push yourself to do heavy housework and shopping. You will certainly need help to start with. It's more a matter of trying as soon as you feel able, and lifting in the correct way.

To lift a heavy object off the ground, you should get as close to it as possible. Bend at the knees into a squatting position, keeping your back straight, or go down on one knee if this is easier. Hold the object close to you and lift it, using the muscles of your arms and shoulders - not your back - then stand up, using your leg muscles. This way you will avoid straining not only your abdominal and pelvic floor muscles, but also the danger of putting your back out. Never bend from the waist and haul the object up, as this will cause strains. And don't lift anything so heavy it really is a struggle.

For the same reasons, it's not sensible to carry heavy shopping (or anything else). When you shop in a supermarket, use a trolley, not a hand basket, unless you are buying only a few light items. Many experts are in favour of everyone using a trolley bag (a shopping bag on wheels) for heavy shopping. There are some more attractive designs available now, so it doesn't have to look geriatric.

If you enjoy gardening, don't do any digging, mowing or hedge cutting until you're fully recovered. Confine yourself to pruning and light weeding. Heavy garden work is notorious anyway for causing hernias and back trouble in perfectly fit people, if it isn't carried out safely, so you always need to be careful.

An abdominal incision will take a couple of months to heal completely and so should not be put under undue stress. And if you had a repair for stress incontinence, this is also a reason not to do anything which causes undue strain. So, although we caution you against excessively strenuous activity, we also encourage you to be as active as possible.

CHAPTER SEVEN
After-Effects

The long-term effects of a myomectomy or hysterectomy should be entirely beneficial, since this is the point of having treatment. In the short term, however, a woman may have problems and anxieties which we can perhaps help to resolve.

Earlier we referred to anxieties about how your sex life will be affected. You will have been advised to wait for about six weeks, until your post-op check-up, following either operation before having intercourse. This allows time for the womb to heal after a myomectomy and, after a hysterectomy, for the incision at the top of the vagina to heal. Your sex life does not have to cease during this time. Lovemaking without penetration is perfectly safe and can also be very reassuring to both partners; it could include caressing, oral sex and mutual masturbation, but couples for whom sex means penetration may need to learn to enjoy these other pleasures. See Further Reading for some helpful sex manuals.

If your relationship with your partner was loving and supportive before the operation, it is likely to be so afterwards. But if you had relationship difficulties, such as a lack of communication and sexual problems, the additional stress of surgery may contribute to these. It is always worth trying professional counselling help, if necessary. Your doctor can put you in touch with a counsellor; see also Useful Addresses.

It will be helpful if we make some general comments on the effects of each operation.

After a Myomectomy

Your womb will have been restored to normal and your fertility preserved by a myomectomy, which is of course the whole point of the operation.

When you restart intercourse, it is unlikely to feel very different to you or your partner, and it may actually have been improved by the operation. The womb is involved in the pleasurable contractions of orgasm and fibroids can interfere with these, so their removal could heighten the sensation. The pelvic floor muscles are also involved in the orgasmic contractions, and so exercising these, as described in the previous chapter, will help to improve orgasm.

Initially, intercourse may be more comfortable if you lie on your side with your partner entering you from behind. An abdominal incision can feel a bit sore and sensitive for a while, and so you may want to avoid positions which put pressure on this area.

Pregnancy

If your main purpose in having a myomectomy was to enable you to become pregnant, you will probably wish to try as soon as possible. You may be advised to wait a minimum of three months, or possibly six, to ensure that the womb has fully healed so you will stand the best possible chance of becoming pregnant. Or it might be considered safe for you to try right away. (It's inadvisable to become pregnant if a myomectomy was combined with surgery for stress incontinence, as it could undo the repair work. But by the time this additional treatment is necessary, a woman is usually of an age when having children would not be a priority.)

A good surgeon will have made the minimum number of incisions into the womb needed to remove the fibroids. This doesn't mean that fewer incisions are always a good thing: several well-placed incisions may actually weaken the wall of the womb less than one or two deep cuts. It depends on the position of the fibroids. But for a woman who wants to become pregnant, the whole point is to preserve as much good wall as possible.

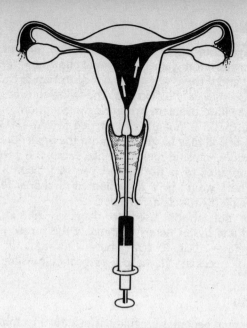

In a hysterosalpingogram (HSG) harmless dye, which can be seen on an X-ray, is injected into the womb and fallopian tubes. Following a myomectomy, it shows whether healing is normal (as here), or if there is still a problem preventing pregnancy. Sometimes HSG helps plan a myomectomy.

The scars from the incisions should not affect your chances of becoming pregnant. Incisions through the full thickness of the womb into the cavity inside must be avoided if possible because the cavity is lined by the endometrium where the embryo will implant. It is obviously better if the cavity can be kept intact for conception and the wall preserved as much as possible for labour.

Should a woman fail to conceive, despite having had fibroids removed which were preventing pregnancy, a hysterosalping-ogram may be carried out. More easily referred to as an HSG, this test is an out-patient procedure. It involves injecting dye into the womb via a slim tube inserted into the cervix. The dye is radio-opaque, which means it will show up on an X-ray (see illustration). If an extensive reconstruction was necessary during a myomectomy, an HSG would show how the womb had healed and if there was any major distortion to the cavity. It would also show any blockage to the fallopian tubes, which can be a separate problem preventing conception.

An anaesthetic is not usually needed for an HSG, but a sedative injection may be given because the procedure can be uncomfortable, causing menstrual-like cramps. It takes from 15 to 30 minutes to perform, and you may need a day to recover. There would be a dye-coloured discharge for a few days and sanitary towels are needed.

HSG is not always used to diagnose fibroids, since ultrasound and hysteroscopy can enable the surgeon to plan a myomectomy, but it may show afterwards if further treatment is necessary to make a pregnancy possible.

Childbirth

When a woman becomes pregnant after a myomectomy, there is a possibility of the womb rupturing during labour. This could happen if an incision made during the operation extended through its full thickness into the cavity to remove a submucous fibroid. (A rupture is highly unlikely to occur during pregnancy.) In this situation a Caesarean birth is usual: the baby is delivered via an abdominal incision.

An attempt at a normal delivery would be allowed under certain other circumstances, if the woman particularly wanted a natural birth. This would be the case if small submucous fibroids had been removed by hysteroscope (see chapter 5). If intramural fibroids within the muscular wall, or subserous fibroids growing out into the abdomen, were the only ones removed during a myomectomy, then the obstetrician may also allow a normal labour to proceed. (An obstetrician is the specialist doctor who manages the pregnancy and birth. In the UK, obstetricians are also gynaecologists.)

The woman's condition during labour would be monitored very closely in hospital for any signs of a rupture, which would then necessitate a Caesarean. Certainly a home birth wouldn't be possible.

A Caesarean can be a fulfilling experience too. Most

planned Caesareans are carried out under an epidural anaesthetic (an injection into the spine; see p 70), which deadens all pain below the waist, and is often used in normal childbirth. You are conscious throughout and, all being well, will be given your baby to hold soon after the birth. Sometimes a general anaesthetic is used if circumstances call for it, or the woman doesn't want to be conscious during the procedure.

If you opt for an epidural, it may be possible for your partner to be present at the birth, should you and he wish it. But he needs to be aware that a Caesarean is a major procedure. Having another person present in the operating theatre is not always an advantage, though; it depends on your obstetrician.

With an epidural, you will not have the after-effects of a general anaesthetic. In other respects, recovery from a Caesarean is very much the same as from any other major abdominal operation, such as a myomectomy; you must allow for the fact that you will also have a baby to look after, so ensure you have enough help.

Should you wish to have more than one child after a myomectomy, it is usually possible. If you've not had problems giving birth either naturally or by Caesarean, then you're less likely to have difficulties with another birth.

Recurrence of Fibroids

A woman who has had a myomectomy will be concerned about whether fibroids are likely to recur. There does seem to be a fairly high recurrence rate, although the fibroids do not necessarily become large or troublesome. About 50 per cent of women who've had fibroids removed develop them again. This may be because there is a natural tendency for fibroids to recur in women who've already had them. Or it may be because not all surgeons remove every fibroid during a myomectomy. There is not sufficient evidence to say definitely which is the case.

Large and troublesome fibroids should always be removed, but small ones may sometimes be left, and it is these which might grow after a myomectomy. If you want to be certain that all fibroids, whatever their size and position, are removed you should definitely request that this be done. The surgeon may do it anyway without needing to be asked, but you may want to be sure.

Recurrence may also depend on the age of the woman when the myomectomy was carried out. The nearer the woman is to the menopause, the less likely fibroids are to recur. A woman who has had a recurrence of troublesome fibroids would most likely be advised to have a hysterectomy, rather than another myomectomy. However, a sympathetic surgeon may well be prepared to perform a further myomectomy. As Professor Campbell says, 'I don't rule anything out. If a woman still has a strong psychological need to retain her womb, and would rather have another myomectomy, I'd do one. You're treating the woman, not just her fibroids.'

After a Hysterectomy

A woman may have a number of anxieties following a hysterectomy and so we will comment on those which are likely to be most worrying. Fortunately, there are also some good books on hysterectomy which do much to dispel the myths and misinformation which have surrounded this operation (see Further Reading).

Women can worry that their partner will find them less attractive without a womb. This is rarely the case. Probably the major anxieties which you both may have about restarting your sex life will be whether intercourse will hurt you and cause any damage to the scar at the top of the vagina. Intercourse shouldn't hurt once healing is complete, although if you've had an abdominal hysterectomy, you may need to find positions to start with where your partner's full weight is not on the incision (see p 84 for advice). Nor is there any danger of damaging the scar in the vagina. If there is a little bleeding initially after sex, this is probably because small granules of tissue have formed around the scar. This is quite common and a doctor can remove them easily and painlessly.

Another worry may be whether intercourse will feel different without a womb. Sexual sensation for both men and women tends to be centred more around the vaginal entrance than deep inside, and so most couples don't notice that the cervix has gone. It's worth saying that some women enjoy having the scar at the top of vagina stretched during intercourse, so taking away the cervix may actually be an erotic advantage.

You may find that the 'tightening up' of the pelvic floor during surgery increases sexual pleasure. Exercising the pelvic floor muscles (see p 79) will restore sensitivity which may have been affected by surgery. It will also help in arousal. If you have difficulty in responding and having orgasms, this is unlikely to have a physical cause related to surgery. The clitoris is the 'trigger' for orgasm. This small protuberance is situated above the urethral opening and is unaffected by the operation. Stimulation by hand or through close body contact during intercourse will still bring about orgasm. It may feel different, however, because the womb is no longer there to contract. Some women say the sensation is sharper.

As explained in the previous chapter, it shouldn't be necessary to remove the ovaries during a hysterectomy for fibroids, except in a small minority of women. Removal of the ovaries, with their hormone supply, can result in vaginal dryness and loss of libido in a pre-menopausal woman, making HRT necessary. When the ovaries remain, you should not have these problems. But if either of you has fears about sex following hysterectomy, lack of desire is often the result, which is why reassurance can be so necessary. Involve your partner, if possible, in the decision to have a hysterectomy, so that any fears he may have can be resolved.

Back to Normal

When you have fully recovered from a total hysterectomy, you won't be aware of any significant physical differences. Leaving the ovaries during a hysterectomy means that, technically at least, a woman remains fertile and so is protected from the menopausal problems due to lack of oestrogen.

It is partly these problems which have given hysterectomy a bad name, and made women fear that they will be left feeling physically below par, prematurely old and depressed. These fears may also derive from the ancient Greek myth that women's emotions originate in the womb so any problems with this female organ are therefore going to make its owner morbid and hysterical (it's easy to see that this word comes from 'hystera', the Greek for womb). The fact is that even when the ovaries have been removed, HRT means that many women today need not experience a premature menopause.

To guard against menopausal symptoms occurring after removal of the ovaries, some gynaecologists insert a hormone implant during a hysterectomy. But HRT may not be prescribed until symptoms occur after the operation. Even then, some doctors may want to wait and see how serious the symptoms are and if they settle down without treatment. There are still doctors who have reservations about giving HRT at all. A woman who has severe symptoms and is not receiving help should see her gynaecologist, or go to a 'well woman' clinic or the menopause clinic of a hospital, where her case will be fully assessed (see also Useful Addresses).

When the ovaries remain, the menstrual cycle continues, but without periods, since the womb has gone. The ovaries will go on producing a monthly egg (ovulation), although of course you can't become pregnant without a womb. The eggs are harmlessly reabsorbed by the body, since they have nowhere to go after a hysterectomy, so there is no 'egg mountain' building up!

All the physical sensations of the cycle will also continue. If, for instance, a woman has mid-cycle ovulation pain and breast tenderness before a period, she will continue to experience them. She will eventually go through a natural menopause (it is another myth that the ovaries fail much earlier after a hysterectomy). At the menopause, however, there won't be the menstrual symptoms of irregular periods and periods ceasing. HRT may be given then, if necessary, to relieve any unpleasant menopausal symptoms which occur.

In conclusion, the evidence is that women who've had a total hysterectomy for fibroids are very often thankful that they no longer have period problems or need contraception. And they can never be troubled by fibroids again. The perfect example of this positive attitude is Rosemary Conley, the British author whose bestsellers on diet and fitness have done so much to promote healthier living. Now in her forties, with a teenage daughter, this is how she views her operation:

'The hysterectomy 13 years ago was the best thing I've ever had. I'd recommend it to anyone, though I kept my ovaries and I do think that's an advantage. No more monthly problems or any of the inconvenience that creates. I certainly feel much better for it. All this talk about the operation making you prematurely old and fat is absolute rubbish.

'Originally, I went to the doctor because I had a fibroid, said I'd like to be sterilized. "Well," he said, "we've had various problems with your womb over the years. If you don't want any more children, let's get rid of it." And I said "Fine."

'It's true I didn't feel 100 per cent for a year. Yet I was taking exercise classes after six weeks. And at first your stomach does blow up like a balloon by the evening. But that disappears as you become fitter.'

CHAPTER EIGHT
New Developments

Encouraging new surgical techniques for treating fibroids are coming into use at the time of writing. Although not yet widely available in many countries, they are worth knowing about in case they are offered to you.

The established techniques which we have described continue to provide very effective treatment for fibroids. These new developments have a number of advantages for the patient, however. When they are used to carry out a myomectomy or hysterectomy, less time is spent in hospital and recovery is faster.

You may have heard the terms 'minimally invasive' or 'key-hole' surgery, so called because the surgeon operates through tiny incisions in the abdomen. Considerable skill is required when operating inside a confined space; it can mean that a myomectomy or hysterectomy takes longer to perform, but this is balanced by the benefits to the patient. Because an abdominal incision is no longer needed, it turns these major operations into relatively minor procedures for the patient. Healing is much quicker afterwards and the scars are scarcely noticeable.

This surgery has been made possible by advances in laser and electrodiathermy techniques, used together with a laparoscope. We'll recap on what these techniques involve. A laser produces a high energy beam of light which is used for cutting, and which seals at the same time. Electrodiathermy uses a wire heated by electric current for cutting; it also seals as it cuts. With both techniques bleeding is therefore much reduced and so, too, are the risks of post-operative complications, such as infection.

A laparoscope, already mentioned in connection with endometriosis (p 40), is a viewing instrument only about 1 cm (½ in) wide with a light and a lens at one end. It enables the surgeon to see inside the abdomen without cutting it open, and was previously used more in diagnosis than surgery.

Laparoscopy is carried out under general anaesthetic in hospital. The abdomen is first inflated with harmless carbon dioxide gas, introduced via a fine needle; the gas pushes the pelvic organs away from each other, making it easier for the surgeon to see them using the light. In addition, tilting the patient slightly head-down helps to separate the intestines from the pelvic organs. It also makes surgery safer because separating the organs prevents them from being damaged. The laparoscope is then inserted into the abdomen through an incision of no more than 1 cm (½ in), made inside or just below the navel. Instruments used to carry out surgery are then inserted through one or more incisions of about the same size (some may be smaller) lower down in the abdomen near the pubic hairline.

It makes it easier if the woman is not overweight. There can be technical difficulties in performing this precision surgery on the overweight because fat restricts movement of the instruments.

If you were to have this type of surgery, it would most likely be carried out as follows, depending on whether you were having a myomectomy or hysterectomy.

Myomectomy

Your operation would first be mapped out using ultrasound (p 35), hysteroscopy (p 36) and possibly HSG (p 85) to see the fibroids' size and position. For 8-12 weeks prior to the procedure, you would be given GnRH/LHRH analogue drugs to shrink large fibroids and make them easier to remove.

It is technically possible to remove all fibroids. However, due to the length of time this form of surgery takes, it is not suitable for removing multiple fibroids. Removing four fibroids of no more than 10 cm (4 in) in diameter is currently considered to be about the maximum. At present, this surgery tends to be used primarily as a treatment for infertility, although it can be used to treat heavy, prolonged periods in certain cases. Subserous fibroids, which grow from the outer wall of the womb, do not really cause fertility problems, unless they press on the fallopian tubes or are large. These may be left if they don't appear to be affecting fertility. They do not necessarily cause heavy, prolonged periods either, and so likewise may be left alone. Submucous ones growing from the inner wall and distorting the cavity are the major culprits.

Prior to the myomectomy, you might have a procedure called myolysis. This would be carried out 6-8 weeks before the operation, and is used in addition to drugs to shrink fibroids. It is effective for certain subserous fibroids which are more deeply embedded, intramural fibroids within the wall, and submucous ones in the inner wall under the endometrium.

Myolysis is otherwise known as 'laser drilling', which is not as alarming as it sounds; all it means is that holes are made in the fibroids using a laser. The result is that the fibroid's bulk is reduced, it becomes much less embedded in the wall and bulges out more, and so requires less cutting to remove it. Deep incisions through the full thickness of the womb into the cavity may thus be avoidable. If you become pregnant afterwards, this may make a natural birth, rather than a Caesarean, more likely.

Procedures For Myolysis

There are two approaches to performing myolysis. It can be done by laparoscopy (which would also be used later in carrying out the myomectomy). You would be in hospital only overnight for myolysis. The laparoscope is inserted under general anaesthetic, as just described, and the laser lower down in the abdomen; at most three or four small incisions would be needed to carry out the procedure. Subserous and intramural fibroids are then drilled.

Following any procedure using laparoscopy you may have feelings of heaviness and discomfort in your abdomen, due to the gas, but you would need only mild painkillers, such as aspirin or paracetamol. And there may also be 'referred' pain in the shoulders for a short time. There would not be any severe pain due to myolysis itself.

The other method of carrying out myolysis uses a hysteroscope – another viewing instrument also about 1 cm (1/2 in) wide, which is inserted into the womb through the cervix. It has a light and a telescopic lens, but in addition there are channels in it: the surgeon looks down one and surgical instruments, such as a laser, can be inserted down another. We have explained how it is used to remove small submucous fibroids by endometrial ablation and resection (see pp 44-6). It can also be used to carry out myolysis several weeks prior to ablation, which means that larger fibroids can be reduced by drilling and then removed by ablation or resection. As with these procedures, myolysis is usually carried out under general anaesthetic and you would be in hospital for maybe only the day, or possibly overnight.

Because a laser coagulates and seals off blood vessels, there should be very little bleeding from the endometrium after myolysis to submucous fibroids. There is usually no more than a light watery discharge for between one and three weeks afterwards. Minipads, or panty liners, would cope with this. Occasionally, there may be heavier bleeding straight after the procedure, in which case a catheter (a tube) is inserted into the womb via the cervix and a special balloon at the end of the catheter is blown up. Pressure from the balloon stops the bleeding and it is left in place for about four hours.

There is generally little pain from this procedure, although there may be menstrual-like cramps. To guard against this, a local anaesthetic may be injected into the cervix following myolysis, before the woman 'comes round' from the general anaesthetic. The risk of infection after myolysis is negligible. You would be advised to wait until you've had a period before having intercourse.

In the weeks leading up to the myomectomy, while myolysis and/or drug treatment on its own are taking effect, you are likely to experience some menopausal symptoms, due to the drugs, as explained on p 53. These will go away once treatment is discontinued. Although you will very likely be infertile while on them, you and your partner should still continue with contraception, using a barrier method (diaphragm or condom), since you cannot be on the pill while taking an analogue drug.

The Operation

When you have the myomectomy by these new techniques, you will be in hospital for only about 48 hours and should allow two weeks for recovery. This will make organizing your life around the operation much easier, but otherwise preparations for surgery are as advised in chapter 6.

So how are fibroids removed without opening the abdomen? The operation is carried out through two or three small incisions, one on the bikini line and probably one each side, plus the incision in or just below the navel through which the laparoscope is inserted to enable the surgeon to see inside. You don't usually need to remove your pubic hair prior to the procedure, although occasionally you may be asked to remove just the top 1 cm (½ in).

If necessary to restore fertility, subserous and intramural fibroids can be 'shelled out' of their capsules by laser in much the same way as when a scalpel is used. With electrodiathermy, a diathermy 'spoon' does the shelling out. The cavity which remains is then overstitched using soluble sutures. Pedunculated fibroids, which grow out from the wall of the womb into the abdomen on a stalk, can be stapled and then cut off by laser or electrodiathermy. Or they can be lassoed with endoloops – soluble stitches which are drawn tight round the stalk, severing the fibroid from it.

Once the fibroids have been freed, they can be cut up into smaller pieces, if required, using a laser, electrodiathermy or an instrument called a morcellator. This is like a combination of an apple-corer and a pair of scissors. It may be heated and is used in a 'nibbling' manner. The smaller pieces of fibroid may then be placed in a laparoscopic bag, which is inserted into the abdomen via one of the incisions. This prevents any bits of fibroid getting lost. They are removed from the abdomen through the incision, which can be widened a bit if necessary. Large fibroids can also be taken out through an incision made in the vagina, called a colpotomy. This is stitched together afterwards with soluble sutures and so are the abdominal incisions, except for an incision in the navel which may not need to be stitched.

Submucous fibroids under the endometrium, or which

protrude on stalks into the cavity, can be removed by endometrial ablation or resection, using a hysteroscope (see p 44). This could be carried out during a myomectomy for fibroids in other sites. Otherwise, ablation or resection would be used alone if submucous fibroids are the only ones needing to be treated.

Recovery

Following removal of fibroids by either of these routes, you will need a day to recover from the anaesthetic. You are likely to have the usual feelings of drowsiness, thirst and possibly nausea, but you should be able to eat and drink by the same evening. The digestive system seems to recover faster after this surgery, possibly because there is minimal disturbance to the intestines.

You may have a drain (a tube) from one of the incisions to remove any collection of fluid in the pelvis. This would be left in overnight. It is highly unlikely that you would need a catheter to help you urinate. You wouldn't be on a drip to rehydrate you unless you had been very sick from the anaesthetic, or had bled a lot, both of which are unusual following this type of surgery. Similarly, a blood transfusion is rarely needed. Antibiotic cover to prevent any infection after surgery is given routinely. It is injected with the pre-med or the general anaesthetic before the operation.

Painkillers are given either by injection or as tablets after surgery, depending on the severity of the pain, which is usually only a mild discomfort. There may be the usual feelings of heaviness inside following a laparoscopy, and referred pain in the shoulders for a day or two, but you will need only mild painkillers to cope with this once you leave hospital. You'll have no trouble walking, or doing most things, but take it easy when you get home and avoid excessive activity. Do as much as you feel able.

You may wish to try to become pregnant as soon as possible. It is considered safe to resume intercourse after about three weeks. This way of performing a myomectomy is new and there is some divergence of opinion as to how soon it is advisable to become pregnant after surgery. You should be guided by your gynaecologist's advice. The great advantage of this minimally invasive technique, however, is that it allows the least surgery possible to be carried out to enable you to become pregnant.

Hysterectomy

Removal of the whole womb, even when it has become bulky with fibroids, is beginning to be done without opening the abdomen, using the laparoscope instead. The surgeon operates through four or five abdominal incisions, each of no more than 1 cm (½ in) long.

As in a conventional vaginal hysterectomy, the womb is removed through an incision at the top of the vagina. But to reduce its bulk so that it can be taken out this way, it may be cut up into smaller pieces inside the pelvis by laser, electrodiathermy or morcellator. These smaller pieces can then be taken out through the incision. The ovaries can also be removed by this technique, if necessary. And colposuspension or a Kelly repair (stitches to support the neck of the bladder) could be done to relieve stress incontinence.

After the operation, there may be a drain from one of the abdominal incisions, which would be left in overnight. You would be most unlikely to need a catheter, a drip or a blood transfusion. Painkillers are given by injection and then tablets, as after a myomectomy. Antibiotic cover is also given routinely with the pre-med injection or the general anaesthetic.

Recovery

You would be in hospital for about the same length of time as for a myomectomy by laparoscopy, but recovery may take a bit longer. There would be a similar reaction to the anaesthetic and to the gas in the abdomen. Another week for full recovery would probably be necessary, so you could expect to be back to normal after about three weeks. More time is needed for healing after a hysterectomy than a myomectomy. If you are in a relationship, your gynaecologist would advise on when you could restart intercourse. This operation would not have any adverse long-term effects, however.

Hope For The Future

Although these techniques for carrying out a myomectomy or hysterectomy are not yet widely used, they do hold out much hope. The purpose of new developments in medicine is to increase your range of choice, so you shouldn't hesitate to ask about them.

CHAPTER NINE
Self-Help

Since it isn't known why fibroids occur, nor are there any self-help methods definitely known to improve them, a woman with fibroids may feel that she can contribute little to her own well-being: any really effective treatment must be carried out by the medical profession. But there are still worthwhile ways in which a woman can help herself, even though it is not proven that they will necessarily have a direct effect on the fibroids.

As advised throughout this book, you will cope much better with this (or indeed any) health problem if you are calm and relaxed than if you are tense and anxious. In the first place, being calm and collected should enable you to communicate more easily with your doctor and gynaecologist, especially if you are also well-informed by reading this book. Secondly, any surgical treatment you decide to have will seem less of an ordeal. As was said earlier, stress undermines us physically and emotionally, so if you can reduce stress and think positively you will very likely be less sensitive to any pain and your recovery may be quicker.

We have also emphasized the advantages of improving your general health through diet and exercise, particularly before any treatment, and this, too, will be an asset in recovery after surgery. If you are recommended to take drugs to shrink fibroids before a myomectomy, a healthy lifestyle will help you through any menopausal symptoms they may cause.

Diet

We'll start with the most obvious means of self-help: eating for health. There does appear to be a link between high levels of the ovarian hormone oestrogen and the increase in size of fibroids; body fat produces oestrogen independently of the ovaries, so being very overweight may be a contributory factor. It also makes surgery for fibroids more difficult to perform and can increase the risks to the patient. In addition, healing takes longer. And large fibroids may be more likely to recur in the overweight after a myomectomy. The benefits of a healthy diet in these circumstances are obvious.

Whether or not a woman with fibroids is overweight, their most common symptom is heavy, prolonged periods. This can lead to anaemia (iron deficiency), which makes you feel fatigued and depressed. A healthy diet helps to combat these effects.

There is now so much detailed advice available on healthy eating – from government guidelines to popular books and magazines – that we shall simply give some useful pointers relevant to a woman with fibroids. See References and Further Reading for sources of general information.

A diet which is low in fat and sugar, high in fibre and includes plenty of fresh fruit and vegetables, is widely recommended. The energy the body uses, and the amount of food needed to provide it, is measured in calories. The speed at which the body 'burns' calories as energy is called the metabolic rate. Some of us naturally burn calories faster than others, but this is also related to how active we are. As we grow older, our metabolic rate decreases and we may become less active, but continue to eat the same fattening foods. This is therefore when weight gain becomes increasingly likely – at around the age when fibroids may also become a problem for many women.

Some foods provide more calories than others and if they are not used up through activity, the excess is stored as body fat, which is of course why eating too much of certain foods causes weight gain. The worst culprits are sugary foods, such as cakes, cookies, confectionery and canned fruit. These are rich in refined sugar, and so also are many processed foods. The sugar concentration in them is much higher than the natural sugar found in fresh fruit. They are often described as providing 'empty energy' because they have little nutritional value and cause rapid weight gain. It's better to avoid them altogether if you are trying to lose weight.

Alcohol is also high in sugar and low in nutritional value. Women are advised to have no more than a couple of small drinks a day, but not on an empty stomach, and to have at least two 'dry' days a week.

Fats provide about twice as much energy as other foods and so are needed in very limited amounts. Only around 5 per cent of your diet should consist of fats, and as much of this as possible should be unsaturated (non-animal). Use spreads and cooking oil derived from vegetables, seeds and nuts. Avoid fried foods.

About 20 per cent of your diet can be made up of lean meat, especially poultry (cut the fat off meat and remove the skin from poultry: the fat is under the skin), low-fat dairy produce (milk, cheese, yoghurt), fish, peas, beans, lentils and nuts.

Dietary fibre, also know as roughage, is found in the form of cellulose in green vegetables and fruit (best if eaten raw) and in bran, cereals, rice and wholegrain flours. It doesn't give us much energy, but is valuable because it adds bulk to foods, which can help weight loss because it's filling without being fattening. It also aids digestion and prevents constipation. Another drawback of processed and convenience (junk) foods is that they generally contain little fibre. Vegetables, salads and fruit should therefore make up around 55 per cent of your diet. Cereals, brown rice, wholemeal bread and pasta can make up the remaining 20 per cent.

This gives a good balance of the foods needed daily to provide the right proportion of vitamins and minerals, and to maintain a normal weight, without having to count calories. If you have difficulty changing your eating habits, do seek help from your doctor or a nutritionist. If necessary, join a weight control club, where other members will encourage you and applaud your progress. Or you could go to a health farm, if you can afford it. This could help not only in weight loss, but to put you 'back on your feet' after a myomectomy or hysterectomy, if your doctor considers it a good idea for you to go there. A health farm diet is likely to be naturopathic: mainly vegetarian with much of the food eaten raw. It cannot be relied on to reform your eating habits once you get home, however. In the longer term, try to eat a balanced diet consisting of healthy, everyday foods.

Dieting on its own is less effective without adequate exercise. But before we say more about the benefits of exercise, here is some further specific advice about diet which may be of additional help to a woman with fibroids.

- If heavy periods have caused anaemia, foods rich in iron can help to relieve fatigue and depression. These include kidneys, liver, eggs, sardines, wheatgerm, wholemeal bread, spinach and dried fruits.

- Menopausal symptoms - such as hot flushes/flashes, night sweats and vaginal dryness - brought on by drug treatment to shrink fibroids before a myomectomy, may be helped by vitamins B6 and E. Vitamin B6 is found in wholemeal bread, rice, liver, fish, avocados, bananas, green leafy vegetables and carrots. Vitamin E is found in fruit, nuts, olive oil, eggs and cereals. These vitamins are also thought to help relieve menstrual problems and PMT; they may also aid fertility.

- Avoiding or cutting down on tea, coffee, cola drinks and alcohol may relieve mood swings due to drug treatment or PMT.

- Taking evening primrose oil may help to balance hormones and relieve menstrual and menopausal symptoms.

- There is some evidence that healing after surgery can be helped by vitamin C; the same may be true of zinc. Vitamin C is found mainly in citrus fruits and green leafy vegetables. Zinc is found in seafood, beef, carrots, tomatoes, mushrooms, nuts and wholemeal bread.

- A healthy, balanced diet should provide all the nutrients you need under normal circumstances. But with a health disorder, such as fibroids, taking vitamin and mineral supplements may be beneficial, depending on your symptoms and the treatment needed. Consult your doctor about this.

Exercise

A healthy diet, especially if it is intended to help you lose weight, needs to be combined with exercise to be really effective. Exercise maintains your muscular tone, and using your muscles burns up calories as energy. Regular exercise can also raise your metabolic rate, so increasing your calorie burning capacity. When dieting, you lose muscle as well as fat unless you exercise, making it harder to avoid regaining weight.

As advised earlier in the book, being in good shape also has definite advantages if you're having surgery for fibroids. It lessens the trauma of the operation and helps you to heal faster. Exercising the whole body is important in recovery too, and in preventing the weight gain which can so easily happen after a major operation, such as a myomectomy or hysterectomy. Contrary to popular belief, there is no reason why gynaecological surgery in itself should cause weight gain - it's being inactive afterwards which is to blame.

Taking really vigorous exercise, however, may not be sensible or possible if you have large fibroids or are recovering from surgical treatment. We have explained the importance of abdominal and pelvic floor exercises after a myomectomy or hysterectomy (see chapter 6). Gentle 'whole body' exercise is best if you have troublesome fibroids, or are recovering from surgery.

Walking is good gentle exercise and so is cycling. Walk or cycle short distances instead of using the car. Swimming is particularly good because the whole body is supported by water while being exercised, so there is no stress or jarring, but don't jump or dive in to start with after surgery. Gentle stretching exercises improve muscle tone and flexibility. These can be done to music and be learnt in a class, which is more fun. Another advantage of attending a class is that you can gradually build up to more active exercises; start in a 'beginners' class and work towards more 'advanced' levels. See Further Reading for books on exercise and fitness.

Relaxation

As we said at the start of this chapter, being calm and relaxed will enable you to cope better with troublesome fibroids and their treatment.

We have referred to deep breathing as a relaxation technique which can be carried out anywhere. It will reduce your natural stress reaction by slowing your heart rate and lowering your blood pressure, which has a calming effect. Here's how to do it. Keep your back straight, breathe in deeply, filling the lungs, using your diaphragm (the muscle between your chest and abdominal cavity). Breathe out slowly, emptying the lungs. Continue to breathe deeply, slowly and regularly. This is actually how you should always breathe and it prevents the rapid, shallow breathing which results from stress.

Correct breathing control is central to Yoga, one of the most popular 'alternative therapies'. Increasingly, people are finding that these therapies promote a sense of calm which helps them through medical treatment, and with their lives in general. The aim of alternative therapies is indeed to help the person as a whole, which is why they are also called 'holistic' or 'whole person' therapies. The value of using them together with orthodox medical treatments is becoming more widely accepted by both doctors and alternative therapists themselves. This is why these therapies are also described as 'complementary': they complete the range of treatment options.

There are therapies and relaxation techniques in addition to Yoga which could help you if you are having treatment for fibroids (being calm and relaxed may even have a beneficial effect on hormonal balance, and so influence the development of fibroids in the first place). We have mentioned acupuncture, aromatherapy and the positive power of suggestion earlier in the book, and will explain more about them. But there is a wide range of therapies which are of overall benefit and we can only touch on those which are more easily available and could be most useful to a woman with fibroids. Again, see Further Reading for detailed books on complementary therapies.

Your doctor may be able to put you in touch with a therapist, and your hospital may offer some complementary therapies, or have contact with outside therapists. Some doctors, nurses and other health care professionals have also trained in various branches of complementary medicine, and so can help you themselves. Or you can contact the organization which represents those therapies you wish to try (see Useful Addresses). They can recommend the nearest therapist who is a member and therefore bound by the organization's code of practice. This means that he/she will be fully trained and reputable. Complementary therapists should not advise you against having orthodox treatment, nor can they offer a cure. But they can do much by helping you to help yourself. Some of the best known therapies originated in the East, where they are part of a philosophy of life.

Helpful Therapies

YOGA AND MEDITATION

This ancient Indian philosophy combines breathing exercises (pranayama) and postures (asanas) as a preparation for meditation. Yoga is Sanskrit for 'union', its purpose being to create harmony between mind, body and spirit. The breathing exercises calm and relax both mind and body, the postures improve flexibility and muscular control, and meditation completes the therapeutic effect. The aim of meditation is to clear the mind of everyday cares, as well as of any greater anxieties, in order to bring complete inner calm.

To aid meditation, you can focus your mind on a colour, a sound or a positive thought. For instance, Hindu meditation concentrates the mind on sacred words (called mantras). Couéism is a Western form of meditation named after Emile Coué, the nineteenth-century French apothecary. The positive power of suggestion is obvious in his famous phrase, 'Every day, in every way, I am getting better and better'. Repeating these words, and allowing them to permeate the deeper levels of your mind, is intended to stimulate your imagination, so that you 'see' the positive effect. Meditation is not meant to make you consciously use your willpower to help yourself; it acts on the whole being in a gentler, more profound way.

These approaches to relaxation could benefit you before and during treatment for fibroids, and in recovery afterwards. Because Yoga is so popular, you are likely to find a class you can attend in your area. You can learn Yoga, and various ways of meditating, from books and tapes, but a good teacher is invaluable. You can also practise in a group or alone, whichever helps you most.

VISUALIZATION

Your imagination could be of direct help in enabling you to feel positive about treatment for fibroids by means of visualization. It is a form of meditation which involves feeling at one with the images you create in your mind. This can help to resolve fears and aid relaxation.

You could allow an image connected with the problem of fibroids to come into your mind and then imagine something happening to improve that image. The image could be symbolic or quite realistic. For instance, if you are facing a myomectomy, a symbolic image could be of a lumpy piece of clay (a womb with fibroids) being fashioned into a useful and beautiful receptacle. Or you could visualize a womb with fibroids looking much as it really does: rather like a knobbly potato, whereas it should resemble a small, smooth pear. You could imagine it transformed from one shape to the other. Similarly, a hysterectomy could be visualized as form of release.

Any post-operative pain might also be eased by thinking of healing images, which could involve light, warmth or coolness soothing the area. But these are simply suggestions, and you would need to conjure up the images which reassure you.

AUTOGENICS

A further means of reducing stress is called autogenic training. It is another way of achieving complete relaxation by activating your imagination. Autogenics is a form of mind-over-body control, which is achieved by relaxing parts of the body by means of the positive power of suggestion. It involves concentrating on such messages as, 'My arms are heavy and warm, my legs are heavy and relaxed, my heartbeat is slow and regular', ending with 'I am at peace' when your whole body is relaxed.

It could be particularly helpful if you are having tests or treatment for fibroids which require only a local anaesthetic or no anaesthetic. Menopausal symptoms, such as mood swings, headaches or fatigue, due to drug treatment before a myomectomy, could be relieved.

You can learn autogenics from books and tapes, but is widely taught and personal instruction in a class is always better. Once learned, it takes only a few minutes to carry out.

T'AI CHI

As its name suggests, T'ai Chi came from China where it is part of the traditional Chinese way of life. It could best be described as meditation-in-motion. Often performed outdoors, it is a sequence of graceful movements intended to tune you into the universal energy, know as Chi. This, it is supposed, runs through all living things. The movements bring about improved physical balance, promoting an inner calm and raising energy levels, so that the movements become effortless. It can be performed with a partner by joining both hands with each other and alternately pushing and yielding.

The overall therapeutic benefits could help you through drug treatment for fibroids, and to regain your strength after a myomectomy or hysterectomy. Women who suffer from premenstrual syndrome and menstrual problems may also be helped. Because the movements are gentle and flowing, there is no risk of overstressing the body.

T'ai Chi is becoming increasingly popular in the West, and is now widely taught in private classes and adult education colleges.

ACUPUNCTURE

Valuable in relieving stress and pain, acupuncture also came to the West from China, where it has many uses in medicine. In the West, it is gradually becoming recognized in orthodox medicine for its ability to relieve nausea and pain.

Acupuncture is based on the principle of energy flow in the body: health problems are seen as a state of imbalance in this flow. According to ancient Chinese tradition, the universal energy (Chi) flows along lines called meridians. Inserting very fine sterile needles into specific points along the meridians frees the flow and restores the balance. The meridians actually coincide with the main nerve pathways, and the modern scientific view is that 'needling' them intercepts pain messages to the brain, so that no pain is felt.

Medically trained acupuncturists, who may work in some hospitals, adhere to basic needling, which means that treatment simply involves the insertion of needles into the appropriate places. On insertion, you might feel a little pain, or just a pinprick, although some people experience only numbness and others feel nothing at all. The needles may be made to vibrate by applying a mild electric current to them, which makes treatment more effective. You would only feel the vibration. The needles can remain in place from a few minutes to about half an hour. It could be of help in hospital after a myomectomy or a hysterectomy.

If you were treated by a traditional holistic acupuncturist before or after hospital treatment for fibroids, the approach would be comprehensive. It could involve the use of herbs. Counselling would also play a part: your diet, lifestyle and emotional attitudes would also be discussed, to see if they could be improved. Menopausal symptoms due to drugs could be helped by acupuncture, and so might pre-menstrual syndrome and menstrual problems, because the pain-relieving effects bring about relaxation.

Acupressure is a form of acupuncture without needles. It can be a means of self-help because you can learn to treat yourself. Finger pressure is used on the meridians and, like acupuncture, it helps you to feel relaxed and comfortable.

AROMATHERAPY

Essential oils extracted from plants are used in aromatherapy. These can help to relieve fatigue, depression, irritability and anxiety. Some, or even all, of these problems may be induced by heavy, prolonged periods caused by fibroids, or the problems may be due to the drugs used to shrink fibroids. We have mentioned earlier in the book that some nurses may be trained in aromatherapy, and that it can be used post-operatively to help relieve pain and enable patients to sleep better.

The oils can be massaged into the skin, inhaled or used in the bath. Marjoram, rose, lavender and geranium can relieve anxiety, irritability and depression. Fatigue may be helped by rosemary, melissa and sandalwood. And eucalyptus, juniper and bergamot may help in healing.

There are further complementary therapies which your doctor or a therapist may consider appropriate, so do ask about them. Therapists are often trained in more than one therapy and so may be able to help you in a variety of ways.

In conclusion, it is worth commenting on the view which is basic to many complementary therapies: that health problems may arise because of some source of frustration and unhappiness, or an unsatisfactory lifestyle, which causes inner disharmony and so undermines our resistance. Although such a link with fibroids is unproven, these therapies nevertheless encourage a positive state of mind through promoting a sense of well-being. Whether or not fibroids coexist with other problems in life, feeling positive is always an asset in resolving whatever difficulties we experience. Fortunately, there are now very effective ways of treating troublesome fibroids - and the purpose of this book is to help you to benefit from the treatment which is right for you.

References and Further Reading

Myomectomy

Dubuisson, J B, Lecuru, F, Foulot, H, Mandelbrot, L, Aubriot, F X, Mouly, M, 'Myomectomy by laparoscopy: a preliminary report of 43 cases', *Fertility and Sterility*, Vol. 56, No. 5, November 1991

Garry, Ray, 'Laparoscopic alternatives to laparotomy: a new approach to gynaecological surgery', *British Journal of Obstetrics and Gynaecology*, Vol. 99, August 1992

Sutton, Chris, 'Operative laparoscopy', *Current Science*, Vol. 4, 1992

Verkauf, Barry S, 'Myomectomy for fertility enhancement and preservation', *Fertility and Sterility*, Vol. 58, No. 1, July 1992

Hysterectomy

Clark, Jan, *Hysterectomy and the Alternatives*, Virago Press, 1993

Dickson, Anne, and Henriques, Nikki, *Hysterectomy - the Positive Recovery Plan*, Thorsons, 1989

Gorman, Teresa (MP), and Whitehead, Dr Malcolm, *The Amarant Book of Hormone Replacement Therapy*, Pan Books, 1989

Hayman, Suzie, *Hysterectomy - What it is, and How to Cope with it Successfully*, Sheldon Press, 1986

Hufnagel, Dr Vicki, *No More Hysterectomies*, Thorsons, 1990

Webb, Ann, *Experiences of Hysterectomy*, Macdonald
Optima, 1989

Infertility

Anderson, Mary, *Infertility - A Guide for the Anxious
Couple*, Faber & Faber, 1987
Barker, Dr Graham H, *Overcoming Infertility*, Hamlyn, 1990
Gunn, Dr Alexander, *Infertility - A Practical Guide to
Coping*, The Crowood Press, 1988
Hawkridge, Caroline, *Understanding Endometriosis*,
Macdonald Optima, 1989
Neuberg, Roger, *Infertility*, Thorsons, 1991
Tan, S L, and Jacobs, Professor H S, *Infertility - Your
Questions Answered*, McGraw-Hill, 1991
Winston, Professor Robert, *Getting Pregnant*, Anaya, 1989
——, *Infertility - A Sympathetic Approach*, Macdonald
Optima, 1987

Health Guides

Bradford, Nikki, *The Well Woman's Self Help Directory*,
Sidgwick & Jackson, 1990
British Medical Association, *The British Medical Association
Complete Family Health Encyclopedia*, Dorling
Kindersley, 1990
Coltart, Tim, and Smart, Felicity, *The Woman's Guide to
Surgery*, Thorsons, 1992
Grist, Liz, *A Woman's Guide to Alternative Medicine*,
Fontana, 1986
Llewellyn-Jones, Derek, *The A-Z of Women's Health*, Oxford
University Press, 1990
——, *Everywoman, A Gynaecological Guide for Life*, Faber
& Faber, 1989
Melville, Arabella, *Natural Hormone Health*, Thorsons, 1990
Phillips, Angela, and Rakusen, Jill, *The New Our Bodies,
Ourselves*, Penguin, 1989
Westcott, Patsy, *Alternative Health Care for Women*,
Thorsons, 1991

Diet

Conley, Rosemary, *Complete Hip and Thigh Diet*, Arrow
  Books, 1989
——, *Diet and Workout Pack*, Arrow Books, 1991
——, *Eat and Stay Slim*, Arrow Books, 1985
——, *Eat Yourself Slim*, Arrow Books, 1985
——, *Guide to Fat in Food*, Grafton, 1989
——, *Metabolism Booster Diet*, Arrow Books, 1991
Graham, Judy, *Evening Primrose Oil*, Thorsons, 1989
Mayes, Adrienne, *The A-Z of Nutritional Health*, Thorsons,
  1991
Newhouse, Sonia, *The Complete Natural Food Reckoner*,
  Thorsons, 1991
Ridgway, Judy, *Vegetarian Vitality*, Thorsons, 1993

Exercise

Alexander, Tania, *No Sweat Fitness*, Mainstream Publishing,
  1992
Conley, Rosemary, *Inch Loss Programme*, Arrow Books,
  1990
——, *Looking Good, Feeling Great*, Marshall Pickering, 1989
——, *Whole Body Programme*, Arrow Books, 1992
Jackson, Lucy, *Medau: Energy for Life*, Thorsons, 1992
Salzmann, Josh, *Bodyfit*, Thorsons, 1992

Relaxation

Goldsmith, Joel K, *The Art of Meditation*, Thorsons, 1991
Hoffmann, David, *Herbal Stress Control*, Thorsons, 1990
Humphrey, Naomi, *Meditation - The Inner Way*, Thorsons,
  1987
Kenyon, Dr Julian, *Acupressure Techniques*, Thorsons, 1987
Kirsta, Alix, *The Book of Stress Survival*, Unwin Hyman,
  1986
Lewith, George T, *Acupuncture*, Thorsons, 1982
Marcus, Dr Paul, *Thorsons Introductory Guide to
  Acupuncture*, Thorsons, 1991
O'Brien, Paddy, *A Gentler Strength - the Yoga Book for
  Women*, Thorsons, 1991

Page, Michael, *Visualization - The Key to Fulfilment*,
   Thorsons, 1990
Tisserand, Maggie, *Aromatherapy for Women*, Thorsons,
   1990

Sex Manuals

Anand, Margo, *The Art of Sexual Ecstasy*, Thorsons, 1990
Brown, Paul and Faulder, Carolyn, *Treat Yourself to Sex*,
   Penguin, 1989
Cauthery, Dr Philip, and Stanway, Drs Andrew and Penny,
   The Complete Book of Love and Sex, Century, 1986
Kitzinger, Sheila, *Women's Experience of Sex*, Penguin, 1985
Stanway, Dr Andrew, *The Lover's Guide*, Sidgwick &
   Jackson, 1992
Yaffé, Maurice, Fenwick, Elizabeth, and Rosen, Raymond C,
   Sexual Happiness - A Practical Approach, Dorling
   Kindersley, 1986

Useful Addresses

If you are concerned about having fibroids, your doctor, local hospital, 'well woman' or family planning clinic can often provide you with the advice you need. If necessary, they may be able to put you in touch with a hysterectomy support group and a complementary therapist. You can also contact the following organizations for information (although this list cannot be comprehensive).

United Kingdom

COMPLEMENTARY THERAPIES
The Institute for Complementary Medicine
PO Box 194
London SE16 1QZ
Tel: 071-237 5165
Library, information service, referrals
Publishes the *Journal of Complementary Medicine*

HEALTH INFORMATION
Women's Health
52-54 Featherstone Street
London EC1Y 8RT
Tel: 071-251 6580
Puts women in touch with health care organizations throughout the country; publishes a newsletter

118   *Fibroids*

Australia

COMPLEMENTARY THERAPIES
Australian Natural Therapists' Association
PO Box 522
Sutherland
New South Wales 2232
Tel: (02) 521 2063
Provides information, advice and referrals throughout
Australia

HEALTH INFORMATION
Healthsharing Women
318 Little Bourke Street
Melbourne
Victoria 3000
Tel: (03) 663 4457

Women's Health Information Resource Collective
653 Nicholson Street
Carlton North
Victoria 3054
Tel: (03) 387 8702

Women's Health Information Centre
Royal Women's Hospital
132 Grattan Street
Carlton
Victoria 3053
Tel: (03) 344 2007/2199

Canada

COMPLEMENTARY THERAPIES
Acupuncture Foundation of Canada
2 Sheppard Avenue East
1004 North York
Ontario
M2N 5Y7

HEALTH INFORMATION
Vancouver Women's Health Collective
Suite 302
1720 Grant Street
Vancouver, B.C.
V5Y 2Y7
Tel: (604) 255-8285

Women's Health Clinic
3rd Floor
419 Graham Avenue
Winnipeg, Manitoba
R3C 0M3
Tel: (204) 947-1517

New Zealand

COMPLEMENTARY THERAPIES
South Pacific College of Natural Therapeutics (NZ) Inc
PO Box 11311
Ellerslie
Auckland
Tel: (09) 579 4997
Advice and referrals

HEALTH INFORMATION
Federation of Women's Health Councils
PO Box 853
Auckland
Puts women in touch with health care services throughout the
country. Write for information.

Fertility Action
2nd Floor
52 Customs Street
PO Box 4569
Auckland
Tel: (09) 366 0296

South Africa

Medical Association of South Africa
PO Box 20272
Alkantrant
Pretoria 0005
Tel: (12) 47 6101
Information on women's health care resources throughout the
country.

United States

COMPLEMENTARY THERAPIES
The American Foundation of Traditional Chinese Medicine
1280 Columbus Avenue
Suite 302
San Francisco, CA 94133
Tel: (415) 776 0502
Brings together Eastern and Western medicine. Offers
information and treatment.

HEALTH INFORMATION
Center for Medical Consumers
237 Thompson Street
New York, NY 10012
Tel: (212) 674 7105

Endometriosis Association
PO Box 92187
Milwaukee, WI 53202
Tel: (414) 355 2200

Santa Cruz Women's Health Center
250 Locust Street
Santa Cruz, CA 95060
Tel: (408) 427 3500

Resolve
5 Water Street
Arlington, Mass 02174
Tel: (617) 643 2424
Infertility advice and information

Index

Notes and Questions